DISPARATE REMEDIES

Intoxicating Histories

Series Editors: Virginia Berridge and Erika Dyck

Whether on the street, off the shelf, or over the pharmacy counter, interactions with drugs and alcohol are shaped by contested ideas about addiction, healing, pleasure, and vice and their social dimensions. Books in this series explore how people around the world have consumed, created, traded, and regulated psychoactive substances throughout history. The series connects research on legal and illegal drugs and alcohol with diverse areas of historical inquiry, including the histories of medicine, pharmacy, consumption, trade, law, social policy, and popular culture. Its reach is global and includes scholarship on all periods. Intoxicating Histories aims to link these different pasts as well as to inform the present by providing a firmer grasp on contemporary debates and policy issues. We welcome books, whether scholarly monographs or shorter texts for a broad audience focusing on a particular phenomenon or substance, that alter the state of knowledge.

1 Taming Cannabis
Drugs and Empire in Nineteenth-Century France
David A. Guba, Jr

2 Cigarette Nation
Business, Health, and Canadian Smokers, 1930–1975
Daniel J. Robinson

3 Remedicalising Cannabis
Science, Industry, and Drug Policy
Suzanne Taylor

4 Mixing Medicines
The Global Drug Trade and Early Modern Russia
Clare Griffin

5 Drugging France
Mind-Altering Medicine in the Long Nineteenth Century
Sara E. Black

6 Psychedelic New York
A History of LSD in the City
Chris Elcock

7 Disparate Remedies
Making Medicines in Modern India
Nandini Bhattacharya

DISPARATE REMEDIES

Making Medicines in Modern India

NANDINI BHATTACHARYA

McGill-Queen's University Press
Montreal & Kingston • London • Chicago

ISBN 978-0-2280-1752-3 (cloth)
ISBN 978-0-2280-1753-0 (paper)
ISBN 978-0-2280-1789-9 (ePDF)
ISBN 978-0-2280-1790-5 (ePUB)
ISBN 978-0-2280-1860-5 (OA)

Legal deposit third quarter 2023
Bibliothèque nationale du Québec

Printed in Canada on acid-free paper that is 100% ancient forest free (100% post-consumer recycled), processed chlorine free

The open access edition of this book was funded by the Wellcome Trust.

Library and Archives Canada Cataloguing in Publication

Title: Disparate remedies : making medicines in modern India / Nandini Bhattacharya.
Names: Bhattacharya, Nandini (Lecturer in South Asian history and medicine), author.
Series: Intoxicating histories ; 7.
Description: Series statement: Intoxicating histories ; 7 | Includes bibliographical references and index.
Identifiers: Canadiana (print) 20230175740 | Canadiana (ebook) 20230175783 | ISBN 9780228017523 (cloth) | ISBN 9780228017530 (paper) | ISBN 9780228018605 (Open Access) | ISBN 9780228017899 (ePDF) | ISBN 9780228017905 (ePUB)
Subjects: LCSH: Pharmaceutical industry—India—History—19th century. | LCSH: Pharmaceutical industry—India—History—20th century. | LCSH: Generic drugs—India—History—19th century. | LCSH: Generic drugs—India—History—20th century. | LCSH: Pharmacopoeias—India—History—19th century. | LCSH: Pharmacopoeias—India—History—20th century.
Classification: LCC HD9672.I52 B43 2023 | DDC 338.4/761510954—dc23

To my parents,
Saradindu and Subhra Bhattacharya

Contents

Figures and Tables

Figures

Tables

Acknowledgements

This book has been written over several years and I have accumulated many debts during this project. I am grateful to the Wellcome Trust for generously funding the research and to my academic sponsor, professor Steven King, for facilitating the application for the fellowship. I would like to thank the AHRI (University of Dundee) and the Carnegie Trust (Scotland) as well as the Science History Institute (USA), which have supported further research for this project.

I wish to thank the staff at the British Library, (London), National Archives of India (New Delhi), Nehru Memorial Museum and Library (New Delhi) Baroda Record Room (Vadodara), Maharashtra State Archives (Mumbai), and the Wellcome Library (London) for their help and support through several years of research.

I have had the privilege of discussing themes in this book with distinguished scholars who have generously offered insights at various stages of writing, and wish to thank Anne Hardy, Mark Harrison, Saurabh Mishra, Laurence Monnais, David Arnold, Projit Mukharji, John Warner, James Livesey, Jim Mills, Kavita Sivaramakrishnan, and Samiksha Sehrawat for their help. My former colleagues at the University of Dundee have been an immense source of intellectual camaraderie and collegial support. I am especially grateful to Matt Graham who diligently read through and commented on drafts. Alan MacDonald provided friendship and encouragement along with rich discussions on history and cricket. Perry Willson, Graeme Morton, Anja Johansen, Mayra Crowe, Murray Frame, Chris Storrs, and Martine Van Ittersum have all been supportive colleagues. In the past year, my new friends and colleagues at Houston, especially Sue Ferguson, Cihan Yuksel, David McNally, Nancy Young, and Abed Takriti have provided unstinting encouragement. I have benefitted too from discussions and arguments with my students. Among several friends who have offered encouragement through the years of completing this project are Stephen Casper, Anne Gerritsen, Akinobu Takabayashi, Samira Sheikh, and Sami Risk. I am thankful for their continued friendship.

I am very grateful to my brother Biswanath and his family who have been helpful and generous hosts during my trips to India. I am indebted to Pratik, who read and commented on much of this work and has lived through the writing of it. Finally, I wish to thank my parents. When I arrived into the world, they agreed between themselves, placed though they were within in an intensely patriarchal society and family, to allow me the freedoms to read and speak my mind. The consequences have not always been happy for them, and I remain grateful.

DISPARATE REMEDIES

Introduction

Disparate Remedies

Making Medicines in Modern India

The pharmaceuticalisation of India in the nineteenth and twentieth centuries occurred in public places. It involved the availability of a great number of ready-made and packaged therapies and nostrums in every bazaar and fancy retail store. The use and abuse of drugs and therapies were entangled in public debates, nationalist discourses, and medical, scientific, and official circles. Questions of efficacy, contents, purity, or impurity of the materials used engaged the emergent public sphere in colonial India. These were intimately related to the larger concerns of economic nationalism, Indigenous enterprise, cultural nationalism, administrative efficiency in controlling epidemics, and the place of science in modern Indian society. This book analyses how medicines were acquired, produced, quality ascertained, and sold in public spheres of modern India. It spans the late nineteenth to the mid-twentieth century from the time when the demand for pharmaceutical commodities expanded in India, to the point where the continued local manufacture of hormonal, synthetic, and antibiotic pharmaceuticals products seemed secure within the independent nation-state.

The term *pharmaceuticalisation* has been mostly used by sociologists and anthropologists and refers to 'the process by which social, behavioural or bodily conditions are treated, or deemed to be in need of treatment/intervention, with pharmaceuticals by doctors, patients, or both'.[1] More recently historians have borrowed the term to analyse the multifarious ways in which medical consumerism pervaded colonial societies.[2] I will argue that the pharmaceuticalisation needs to be situated historically to see how it embedded the participation of the producers and consumers of the therapeutic products who voiced medical and cultural insights into every contemporary social and political issue in modern India. From their opinion of therapies to accentuate virile masculinity to combat colonial rule to the comparative advantages of meat 'juice' to the Indigenous mixture *Chyavanprash* to aid the concentration of young men studying for examinations in government service, there existed competing consumer products and conflicting opinions for everyone across the political spectrum.

All the above trajectories encompassing Indigenous medical systems and what was referred to as allopathy or, more generally, as the Western medical system, were intensely interlocked in the competition for legitimacy and, even more crucially, for government pecuniary support and patronage. The term *biomedicine* is post-dated in some of the debates; I have, therefore, used the nineteenth-century term *scientific medicine* throughout this book.

In 2005, a few years before I began the research for this book, India was the largest producer of medicines in the world by volume (although not in value), and the biggest manufacturer and exporter of essential drugs and pharmaceuticals to developing nations.[3] Its manufacture of antiretrovirals had helped to stall the deadliness of HIV in Africa, and its production of cheap, generic pharmaceuticals even aided developed nation-states like the UK to sustain its universal health care system. Meanwhile, Ayurveda, one of its Indigenous systems of treatment, had generated products that were an essential component of 'well-being' in the beauty/cosmetics and pharmaceutical industries. Yet the fault lines in this celebratory narrative gaped starkly. The TRIPS agreement in 1995 either stalled the manufacture or hiked the prices of generic drugs many times over within the Indian subcontinent.[4] One prominent firm was found by the USA's FDA to have systematically falsified its data with full knowledge of its senior management.[5] India itself was saturated, it appeared, in locally manufactured counterfeit drugs and pharmaceuticals, and the line between manufacturing generic drugs and counterfeit appeared blurred.[6]

All these generated queries about the antecedents of the pharmaceutical industry in India. Did its spectacular successes represent the policies of the postcolonial nation, uncharacteristically prescient in implementing state policy in this instance? Or was it due to the triumph of private enterprise and strategy, irrespective of awkward government intervention? Perhaps it was due to the emphasis on nationalist scientific and medical research in colonial India. The clue, this book argues, is in understanding the public culture of medicine in India. Medicines were transformed in colonial India, epistemically and materially in public spheres: in markets, nationalist politics, and the burgeoning consumer cultures. If these took specific colonial forms, then we also need to ask how Indian modernity was negotiated through the collection, marketing, prescriptions, and consumption of new and modern medicines. It is from this point that we could, perhaps most urgently, ask if it were possible to retrieve a public culture of medicine for the masses from nationalist discourse and politics to the still unequal postcolonial nation. This is probably also the moment to ponder why and how disparate remedies subsist in contemporary India. Pharmacies in any Indian city will stock generic and branded prescription medicines along with familiar and newly produced branded Ayurvedic ointments and pills, powders and capsules, Unani ointments and oils, and even homeopathic pills. At wholesale spice markets in Bombay or in Calcutta, there are invariably a few traders who specialise in Ayurvedic or in Hakimi drugs, some bottled, the rest dried or minimally processed. Disparate remedies are readily and plentifully available, especially to urban consumers across the Indian subcontinent. Advertisements with graphic images and bold print crowd the public sphere. All of these continue to foster a culture of extensive self-medicalization and pharmaceuticalisation among the public and appear as an entrenched aspect of the culture of consumption.[7]

The Public in Modern India

The historiography of the emergence of public culture in colonial South Asia is rich. Following Jürgen Habermas' celebrated analysis of the creation of the public sphere through print communication in Western liberal democracies, scholars have explored the print cultures of colonial India with its politics. As historians have pointed out, the constitution of the public and the public sphere in modern India was negotiated not only through a reading public but was mediated through older traditions such as public debates and more informally through discussion at public sites such as bazaars and streets.[8] Nonetheless, the explosion of print culture in regional languages enabled the formulation of new social identities variously; of community, language, caste, profession, and trade. Regional and communitarian identities shifted and coalesced; identified their collective agendas and reordered their mythologies, competing and negotiating with the traditional or the emergent hegemonic elite, in tandem with the numeracies and gazetting of the colonial state. In brief, the discourses of Indian nationhood were articulated and conditioned through the constantly negotiated public sphere from the nineteenth century.[9] Public opinion was engendered and circulated through educational institutions, learned societies, voluntary and co-operative organisations, trade associations, and their journals and periodicals.

As Francesca Orsini has pointed out in her study of the formation of the Hindi public sphere in colonial India, this was not invested in the state, its laws, and formulations, unlike in Habermas' understanding of French or more generally, the European public. She argues that this is because the state itself was not perceived by Hindi intellectuals or litterateurs as 'their' state – 'for in an important sense it was not *their* state: thus, they concentrated either on delimiting its sphere of competence, finding spaces for themselves within the state, or with replacing it with an Indian state'.[10] Moreover, as Partha Chatterjee had previously pointed out, the division between 'public' and 'private' spheres enabled the Indian elite to formulate its political identity without exposing its domestic or intimate life to radical disruption.[11]

Vernacular literary worlds in colonial India existed outside the remit of the colonial state.[12] For instance, in western India, the divide between Marathi and English languages and their publics proved to be decisive by the mid-nineteenth century. Therefore, social hierarchies among the Indigenous elites were crystallized by the distinct and 'monolingual' vernacular and the English literate communities, the latter claiming to represent the emergent nation.[13] Vernacular languages themselves were reformulated in the process of being the vehicle for subjective identification with communities and identities.[14]

The significant qualification of most historians who have written on the theme is that the public sphere functioned autonomously to the state in colonial India. In their introduction to the volume on public culture and modernity in India, Breckenridge and Appadurai pointed out that the public 'refer[s] to a set of arenas … that have emerged in a variety of historical conditions and that articulate the space between domestic life and the projects of the nation-state … Public in this usage ceases to have any necessary or predetermined relationship to formal politics, rational communicative action, print capitalism, or the dynamics of the emergence of a literate bourgeoisie. Thus, the term becomes emancipated from any specific Euro-American master narrative and indicates an arena of cultural contestation in which modernity can become a diversely appropriated experience'.[15]

For all the scholarly explorations into the flourishing public sphere in modern India, it is impossible to write the state out altogether. The formation or articulation of the public sphere in modern India has always had to reckon with the state. Every vernacular expression in colonial India engaged with the state and its framework of governance; this is manifest in legitimating vernacular languages within state education, government employment, law courts, and public life. Historians have reflected upon the public sphere while writing on the processes of the standardisation of Hindi, Marathi, and other regional languages. They have reflected that these processes enabled the consolidation of singular religious identities and the renegotiation of communitarian and caste identities in modern India. The discourses in the public sphere in Bengali or Hindi, Tamil and Marathi, similarly facilitated the reification of gender hierarchies and gendered spaces within the domestic home. However, these were all enacted in negotiation with their relationships with the state. The colonial state mediated social relations in multiple contexts: domestic, gender, caste, communal, and the occupational identities of Indians. One of these relationships was even more intimate; it was with the bodies of the colonised.

The point that this book makes about the public spheres of medicine in India is that it is essential to understand how the spaces of public culture in colonial India were *negotiated* with the state. The colonial state remained the largest procurer of drugs in India; it was also its largest distributor. At the same time, it remained the main arbitrator of the various public debates around the efficacy, standardization, and purity of drugs, and the various epistemological traditions. This perception of the negotiation between the public sphere and the state allows us to appreciate the problematic 'adulteration' that dominated the debates in the Indian medical market. Chapter 5 shows that, despite the strong rhetoric from the state and the medical practitioners around adulteration, disparate drugs of different potencies continued to be sold in the market. In the absence of government legislation or an official pharmacopeia, the hierarchy of market prices determined the potency and efficacy of drugs in colonial India.

The Public Spheres of Medicine

The book begins by examining the expansion of the domestic market in finished therapeutic products in nineteenth-century urban India. Initially based on the consumption by British officials and elite Indian consumers, the expansion took place through the institutions of the colonial state, such as the postal service that enabled, printed mailed catalogues, rail networks, as well as the burgeoning urban life and grand galleried retail stores in the colonial port cities. These created a new metropolitan lifestyle that led to the demand for a range of consumer goods including cosmetics, medicated wine, patented medicines, and packaged nostrums. Chapter 1 of this book situates colonial India in the market for therapeutic and related cosmetic commodities in the late Victorian age.

Historians have identified the disjuncture within Indian medical traditions and their subsequent marginalisation through state support for Western medicine. More crucially, a body of research over the previous two decades has highlighted how Ayurveda was reformulated and codified, its praxis widened and redefined, and its position/s relocated in the emergent public sphere in colonial India.[16] A similar trajectory of consolidation occurred among Unani practitioners in modern India who too transformed their medical praxis, training, and relationship with their patients and participated in the Urdu public sphere – in brief, they refashioned their corporate identity.[17] Historians have debated the nature of these responses; whether they were in collaboration with British medical officials or if these trends more truly represented the anti-colonial public sphere.[18]

Others have highlighted that the codification of the high traditions and the consolidation of the corporate bodies of Ayurveda and Unani-Tibb marginalised, excluded, and appropriated selectively from subaltern healing traditions in colonial India.[19] David Hardiman and Projit Mukharji have pointed out how subaltern healing practices and traditions, often bereft of any textual reference, were written out of the modernized and classical medical systems of high tradition such as Ayurveda, Unani-Tibb, and, to an extent, Siddha.[20] The examples of *Chandshi* healing in Bengal and the Pentecostal faith healing that fused with Adivasi cultural norms, replacing traditional healing deities in western India, Mukharji and Hardiman have respectively demonstrated that 'folk' remedies cannot be accommodated within the meta-narratives of the 'classical' medical systems in modern India. Mukharji's exhortation to disdain the reification of any medical system through linear narratives resounds with the historian sensitive to the highly hierarchical Indian society and to the limited, elite place of literacy within it. Nonetheless, historians have persuasively argued for the ability of subaltern medical practitioners to change their practices and codify their values through the public sphere and in negotiation with the state in modern India.[21] Elite, high-caste men did not have a monopoly on Ayurvedic practice in colonial north India; as well as subaltern practitioners, a few women too participated in the public sphere and debated the place of medicine within nationalism.[22] Perhaps not surprisingly, it is anthropologists more than historians who have studied subaltern medical cultures in contemporary India that do not fit into the classical medical systems.[23]

The theme of Indigenous medicine in modern India has engaged historians to think in terms of cultural 'encounters' and conflict, but also of reformulating traditions and processes of negotiation and transformation of their institutions, practices, and identities in negotiation with scientific medicine and occasionally in defiance of it. Mukharji has argued that a class of medical practitioners emerged who 'vernacularized' Western medicine, particularly in Bengal where the first medical colleges were established. He has demonstrated how Western medical knowledge and practice were refashioned in historical, Indigenous contexts by Indian practitioners known as *daktars*, a differentiated group, and argues that their medical practice and participation in the Bengali public sphere made Western medicine 'vernacular' as well as 'nationalist'.[24]

In a detailed study of family-run manufacturing firms of homeopathic medicines in colonial Bengal, Shinjini Das has similarly discussed how homeopathy, a German heterodoxy, was translated (in text and in public discourse), made familiar, and popularised within popular culture in India at this time. [25] Das too has interpreted this popularising as an instance of vernacularizing of Western medicine. I suggest that Ayurveda, homeopathy, and even mainstream 'Western' medicine itself were vernacularized in modern India. Das situates homeopathy as a vernacular regime of praxis in colonial India. I suggest that *all* Western medical traditions were culturally appropriated and translated in text and praxis in colonial Bengal, and most explicitly by the upper-caste Hindu elite because they were best placed to access as well as translate these textually and culturally for ordinary Bengalis.

It was not only homeopathy that was vernacularized. In the nineteenth century, the entire spectrum of what is commonly referred to as 'Western medicine' entertained therapeutic heterodox trajectories that included mesmerism, hydrotherapy, naturopathy, osteopathy, and chiropractic practices and even more numerous, albeit transient, trends that included hypnotism and alcohol therapy.[26] Therefore, the translation or interpretation of Western medical traditions, conventional or heterodox, and their cultural appropriation by the educated classes is not unexpected, exceptional, or even uniquely colonial. The crucial question here is, how did they prevail or create spaces within a crowded medical marketplace, and how, and if at all, did the medical establishment accommodate these?

This brings us to the question of the state in the public spheres of medicine in India; did it intervene with the practise of these heterodoxies? The 'braiding' that Mukharji refers to in his recent book of commodities of Western technologies – such as the watch, the stethoscope, and the microscope, selectively with compatible Ayurvedic norms, rituals, cosmological schema to refashion Bengali Ayurvedic (or 'ayurbed') praxis – offers insights into the dynamism of the high tradition in Bengali Ayurveda. However, it does not engage with the state.[27] Yet, every therapeutic reinvention in Indigenous medical traditions was directed at the state as well as the public. Their copious textual testimonies in the Bengali medical and lay press (as well as, it must be added, in the English press in India) were in dialogue with the public *and* with the government. In colonial India, where representative politics was negligible, these represented discrete elements; official and medical discourse often conflicted with public discourse on health policy. Indigenous medical practitioner's wanted, above all, validation from the state so that the members of their now professional bodies could access government employment and legitimately offer expert medical advice in the official business of government. They wanted their therapeutic remedies prescribed in government dispensaries. They might translate European heterodoxies or refashion Western technologies to enhance their everyday medical praxis and disseminate these in their own language/s, inviting public approval and custom. However, they were also acutely aware that the clearest visibility of their therapeutic regimes would be through legitimacy by the state, through legislation, or at least administrative approval. For example, Kavita Sivaramakrishnan has studied how Ayurvedic practitioners reinvented themselves in Punjab and northern India. They organised themselves into professional bodies, established medical schools and dispensaries, popularised their therapies in print, and marketed their medicines in modern packaging through bottles and pills. They articulated their causes, which included the demand for legitimacy from the government in the public sphere and participated in nationalist politics of multiple hues. Similarly, Rachel Berger has pointed out how Ayurvedic practitioners in late colonial north India argued for the legitimacy of their praxis, lobbied for government support and employment, and presented themselves and their knowledge as the repository of both textual and practised ancient and modern Indian (which they interpreted as essentially Hindu and Sanskritic) knowledge.[28] Berger argues for validation of Ayurveda practitioners by the provincial Congress government in Upper Provinces in 1937–39, when it tried to pass legislation on Indigenous systems of medicine and allowed limited employment of Ayurvedic physicians within the provincial dispensaries. Nonetheless, despite the Congress government's sympathy towards Indigenous medical practitioners, the validation of even Ayurveda (and concurrent exclusion of Unani and Hakims) by the government remained limited. Similarly, A. Cerulli highlighted how Indigenous medical practitioners lobbied the government to validate their modern, integrative curricula and the degrees offered in their new colleges from the late nineteenth century.[29] The public sphere, medical praxis, and the state were intimately connected in colonial India. Chapter 2 of this book shows that the emergence and establishment of new Indigenous laboratory-based pharmaceutical companies were directly connected to the patronage they received from either the colonial government or the provincial princely states. The firms straddled nationalist support for Indigenous production and colonial investment in medical institutions simultaneously, using the public sphere such as nationalist discourse, print, and the logic of Swadeshi to negotiate favourable terms for their commodities. Chapter 4 argues that the government itself manufactured and distributed medicines at a profit to civil institutions, and its Medical Store Department could significantly influence the prices and availability of drugs in the medical market.

State Medicine in Colonial India

The history of public health in modern India has engaged scholars deeply as the site of negotiation between the state and the public (and their colonised bodies). As David Arnold has pointed out in his study of the pandemics of cholera, smallpox, and plague in nineteenth-century British India, epidemics were sites of intense conflict. In fact, the processes of implementing vaccination and sanitary programmes for cholera and smallpox (and the episodic use of the military in enforcing quarantine in western India) became an integral part of the consolidation of the colonial state's authority.[30] Yet the arm-to-arm transmission of the smallpox vaccine or the use of forcible segregation and quarantine during the plague epidemic were episodic and transient experiences for most Indians. The oppressive state policies in western India during the plague engendered a ferocious backlash and aroused nationalists of multiple hues to protest through armed violence as well as insurgent editorialising in the nationalist press. In the longer term, the government's sanitarian and vaccination policies were attenuated in both policy and praxis. For instance, as Saurabh Mishra has demonstrated, the imperial policies to control cholera epidemics transmitted through Indian Haj pilgrims at Mecca were mediated by the competing authorities of local governments, the Urdu press and intelligentsia, and colonial anxieties about interfering drastically at religious events.[31] Even in the context of the greater imperial significance of the plague, local politics and exigencies tempered the government's response in Bombay.[32]

Outside the metropolitan port cities and hill stations, state interventions were only orchestrated at the time of infectious epidemics.[33] As Mark Harrison has demonstrated, even in the capital city of Calcutta, it was difficult to sustain a municipal government that would prioritise investment in public health infrastructure.[34] Harrison has argued that this neglect was the consequence of the local elites' resistance to municipal taxes to fund expensive sanitation and piped water systems in the late nineteenth century. Similarly, the expensive drainage systems and conservancy works carried out in mid-nineteenth-century Bombay were toned down by the newly instituted municipality (legislated for in 1872) once it was given jurisdiction over the expenditure on public health.[35] Indeed, historians of colonial India have reflected extensively on the low investment in public health by the colonial state and wondered alternatively if it were the Indigenous elite that did not value sanitary policies and civic urbanism; or at least, not in the image of their manifest forms in Victorian Britain.[36]

Nonetheless, the implementation of medical policies by the state touched the everyday lives of most Indians to varying degrees. The associated fears of miscegenation, the high mortality rates in the army from sexually transmitted diseases, and more broadly, a puritanical suspicion of corporeal pleasure induced the Contagious Diseases Act and the Venereal Diseases Act in India (as in Britain and indeed, in the British Empire generally) from the mid-nineteenth century.[37] As scholars have demonstrated, these Acts identified Indian women (many, but not all, of them prostitutes) who were intimate with British soldiers as the sites of sexual diseases and their transmission, and policing their bodies was, therefore, one of the first ways that Indians received therapeutic treatment from British medical personnel. This was, of course, apart from the Indian troops who were treated under the supervision of British surgeons in the Company's army.[38] While the cholera epidemics of the nineteenth century within India did not provoke the large-scale interventionist policies by the government, they elicited close encounters between British medical and administrative officials and missionaries and Indian religious rituals and sanitary norms beyond the cities, in the deep interiors of the subcontinent.[39] The conservative Indian Medical Service (IMS) and an administration that was scarred by the memories of the armed 1857 revolt agreed that cholera was not contagious through person-to-person contact. The anti-contagionists in British India, therefore, favoured policy that did not require drastic intervention to control the mass movement of people, not even in crowded religious festivals or long pilgrimages across the subcontinent. This view was challenged internationally by medical research and by several European powers. The contagion–anti-contagion debate on the epidemiology of cholera remained richly contentious in medical discourse and informed international diplomacy until the turn of the nineteenth century. The countervailing theories of the epidemiology of cholera have intrigued historians of South Asia, as well as Britain, and occasioned debate as polarising as the medical theories themselves.[40] Nonetheless, when the elite in colonial society were endangered, or public health was compromised to the point of disruption of international commerce, coercive sanitary and medical interventions were available and used unequivocally by the state. Finally, when the unclaimed dead were dissected in the morgues, Indian bodies encountered the colonial state and its medical praxis intimately.[41]

These processes served to entrench and negotiate the relationship between the growing Indian middle class and the state. The emergent public in colonial India engaged with the state, and not only at the time of epidemics or death. Although historians have little noticed it, emergent nationalist politics engaged deeply with the state at the sites of the use and abuse of medical therapies, both Western and Indigenous.

Scientific Medicine and the Public in Colonial India

The urban poor and even the emergent middle classes had to take notice of the state and its interventions for sustaining sanitary cordons for the ruling elite during pandemic outbreaks, such as the plague in Bombay in the 1890s. Even beyond the remits of surveillance and coercion, public health and epidemiological obfuscation, there were other, less contentious sites where Indians could experience Western medical therapies in their everyday lives. These were in the Western-style hospitals and dispensaries. The hospital system in British India emerged from the military hospitals for the troops of the East India Company. These were extended to civilian populations in the colonial port cities; first to Europeans and then to Indians as well by the middle of the nineteenth century. These institutions disseminated 'scientific medicine', as its proponents called it, to Indians more widely. Mark Harrison has pointed out, quite correctly, that although the colonial government supported Western-style hospitals; their establishment did not necessarily represent a singular journey towards modernisation, instead incorporating in their medical practices elements from local medical cultures.[42] Nonetheless, the colonial hospital (and not only lock hospitals and lunatic asylums) represented a disjuncture between Indigenous medical practices and Western medicine, which distinctively provided a gateway to scientific and new medicine through medical training, the use of scientific instruments such as stethoscopes and thermometers, and a more thorough knowledge of anatomy and surgery through the dissection of corpses.[43] In turn, the hospitals used local men and women of low castes as manual and sanitary labourers and provided medical training to high-caste aspirants for supplementary and subordinate medical tasks such as compounding prescriptions, thereby cementing and enhancing the institution of castes in Indian society. [44] As Pratik Chakrabarti has argued, colonial hospitals were not merely the sites of modern and scientific praxis and representing the new imperial power, they were also the sites of the colonising process itself and of its concomitant experiences.[45] Indeed, this is clear enough when we see how scholarship on colonial India has linked the extension of scientific medicine with the colonial state's attempts to access gendered spaces in the nineteenth century.[46] This occurred through the Countess Dufferin Fund's women physicians who treated veiled upper-caste women in the zenanas, or the specialised training for the untrained and unsanitary dais (midwives) to attend childbirth in rural areas.[47] Even medical missionaries at the Christian hospitals, which mostly served marginalised and isolated communities, were sustained by the discourse of the scientific modernity of their medicine.[48]

In official medical discourse, this scientific modernity was placed in contestation with the 'empiricism' of the Indigenous medical traditions. Modern Western medicine was deemed scientific, whereas the use of most Indigenous drugs was held by Western medical experts to be 'empirical', i.e., based on hearsay, text, or use, without knowledge of the drug's constituent properties. Even advocates of using Indigenous drugs in British India referred to Ayurveda or Unani as 'empirical systems'.[49]

Meanwhile, Western medical therapeutic principles and practices had transformed fundamentally in the mid-nineteenth century, incorporating fixed, general norms for human physiology instead of the traditional approach of treating each patient's body as distinctive.[50] In the West, the professional medical associations, hospitals and their medical colleges, and manufacturing/research laboratories now shared authority over therapeutic practices and over the bodies of citizens or subjects, along with the state. The medical marketplace here, although still crowded with informal therapies, secret remedies, and illegal 'quacks' was, nonetheless, formalised. Many occupations offering medical services – doctors, surgeons, nurses, dentists, and apothecaries – were organised into professional bodies with self-regulating norms and formal training regimes in place. Other trades, such as herbalists or corn cutters faded away with industrialisation and through competition from the stronger, legitimised medical occupations. Although these processes were gradual and took place throughout the nineteenth century, they represented to the British, along with the industrial production of therapeutic products, a different and superior form of the medical system from the therapeutic practises of Indian medical practitioners of all classes and knowledge systems. The confrontation between scientific, Western medicine, and Indigenous medicine occurred in the context of colonisation and the evident favour with which the state treated the exponents of Western medicine. When the government withdrew the modestly funded native medical institutions in Calcutta in 1833, it spelled the end of any institutional accommodation with Indigenous systems of medicine, as indeed with the Orientalist vision of recasting Indian institutions in their ancient golden age.

The modern military and civilian hospitals and teaching colleges practised and trained Indian students in the new scientific medicine, where anatomy and surgery featured distinctively.[51] The hospitals, clinics, and dispensaries were the preferred means by which the government sought to extend Western medicine in the late nineteenth century. In a typical illustration of colonial administrative priority and parsimony, the government encouraged local philanthropy to establish and support hospitals and dispensaries, especially in the districts and mofussils.[52] The local government supported these with grants and loans from time to time, and the Indian army provided the personnel to run the government hospitals in the presidency capitals and prominent district headquarters.[53] The hospitals and dispensaries were at the forefront of vaccinations and surgical treatment and provided outpatient treatments for everyday medical care. The hospitals were also the sites where the therapeutic remedies of Western medicine were prescribed to poorer Indians and in cities as well as mofussil towns.

Apart from the single exception of 'pice-packets' (each packet costing one pice, the smallest monetary unit in British India denoted by a coin) of quinine distributed through post offices to areas of endemic malaria, the charitable dispensaries were the most likely sites where common Indians had access to Western medicine products.[54] Although scholars have written histories of Indian hospitals and medical colleges, these have (as above) largely focussed on their status as state-supported or, alternatively, philanthropic institutions. Pratik Chakrabarti has argued for eighteenth-century hospitals in British

India as the sites of collection and appropriation of local medicines, but historians have not thought of colonial hospitals as the sites of popularising Western medical therapies. Even the medical officials who published accounts of their more interesting medical cases in professional journals referred most often to surgical cases. Yet the hospitals requisitioned dozens of Western therapies, bottled or in tablet form, in powders, mixtures, or in concentrated form for use through injections. Some of these came from the Indian army, some were manufactured in-house in the army's medical stores, and others were imported from British firms by the army and sold at a profit to the hospitals and dispensaries. One of the incentives offered to establish and maintain charitable dispensaries and hospitals in British and India in the nineteenth century was the assurance of a supply of medicines from the army stores. In addition, hospitals and dispensaries emerged as significant customers of medical therapies from the government and, eventually, the private market.

It is important to locate this history of dispensaries and hospitals as harbingers of 'scientific medicine' within the wider backdrop of the modes of procurement and distribution of drugs in British India. As chapter 4 shows, the Government Medical Store, which was part of the Indian army, controlled the cultivation, manufacture, and much of the distribution of drugs. It was a lucrative organisation of the state with profits that were generated through the sale of drugs at controlled prices and regulated supply to civil institutions.

Disparate Remedies

The principal themes that resonate with the practice of medicine in colonial India have been the institutionalisation of scientific (or Western) medicine, the changing practices and consolidation of Indigenous medical traditions, and, finally, the state-supported institutions of scientific medicine and their conflict/negotiations with Indigenous medical systems. Several scholars have probed closely and challenged the binaries of conflict or the trope of 'encounter' to instead posit a more nuanced approach that acknowledges the dynamism of Indigenous medical traditions. They have demonstrated how their practitioners took the opportunities made available to them to reinvent themselves and their craft, enter into dialogue with Western medicine, and participate in the public sphere and nationalist politics in colonial India. The studies have been focussed on changing professions, or institutions, and have remained distinct from the histories of drugs themselves.[55]

Historians have demonstrated how apothecaries in Britain and Holland experienced manifold increases in the variety and the quantities of drugs and medicines available to them through the expansion of global commerce from the seventeenth century.[56] By the nineteenth century, imperial commercial networks enabled not just the Apothecaries Society in Britain, but individual manufacturing and trading companies to produce and export their goods.[57]

The vast extension in Western apothecaries' repertoires through global commerce was facilitated by the European ships' surgeons who often had to rely on local materia medica in the East or the West Indies.[58] Europeans were introduced to Indian medical therapies and practices predominantly through the use of drugs from the local bazaars and encounters with local medical men, collectors, and their interlocutors, and incorporated these practices, shorn of their cultural contexts, through a process of appropriation and analytical contraction.[59] Generally historians of drugs in the Indian subcontinent have studied the circulation of single drugs across multiple trading networks, political borders, and epistemological boundaries and have shown how their nomenclature, uses, and identities changed in the process.[60]

Yet in the late nineteenth-century India, along with South Africa and Australia, there was a large market for industrial pharmaceutical commodities, including drugs, branded therapies and cosmetics, and patent medicines from Britain and the USA.[61] Its consumers were the affluent mercantile and landed classes as well as a large emergent professional middle class who lived in its burgeoning cities and towns. The colonial consuming public was differentiated and heterogeneous and occupied a prominent place in its public culture. They had a choice from a vast range of medicines at the market. Imported therapeutic products were sold alongside locally manufactured therapies that varied in price, quality, and processing and packaging techniques. In the late nineteenth century, everyone, from an itinerant peddler to a distinguished fifth-generation Ayurvedic or Hakimi practitioner, a 'compounder' or a dispenser trained on the job to a British-qualified pharmacist and distributor of imported remedies, could sell medicines. Anyone who could source drugs and spices and knew formulae, whether the knowledge had been obtained from official and published pharmacopeia or entirely from witnessing them being prepared, produced drugs for the market. The government, itself, sourced and produced a large number of drugs and therapeutic products that it distributed to the government and aided hospitals at profit.

Such a disparate medical culture also provoked acute anxiety about the availability, efficacy, and quality of the drugs in the market. To some extent, the anxiety about the scarcity of drugs was secondary to the concern about their high prices or poor quality. Medical and popular discourse decried the abundance of poor-quality medicines in the market and debated the reasons for this. Explanations abounded; while official medical discourse pointed the finger at the dubious practices of Indian 'bazaar traders' as well as manufacturers of Indigenous medicines, popular opinion was more divided and blamed all traders and most manufacturers. Ayurvedic and Unani practitioners, as well as many local manufacturers of Indigenous and Western medical therapies, popularised the view that only Indigenous or locally grown and produced therapies were suitable for Indian bodies. Distributors of imported medicines, whether British or 'bazaar traders', pointed out that imported and branded medicines adhered to the standardised British Pharmacopeia (henceforth BP) and were, therefore, above reproach. These intensely debated points were relevant to the very legitimacy of either 'Western' or Indigenous epistemologies, their texts, or their pedagogic practices.[62]

In fact, as chapter 3 of this book shows, these public debates of standards and purity were fundamental because while the modes of processing them differed, as well as the rhetoric of their respective heritages, the difference between Indigenous therapies and so-called scientific drugs in terms of their ingredients or their efficacy remained indeterminable. The drugs used for curative purposes remained broadly similar in Indigenous and Western medical treatment and were of similar botanical/mineral/animal origins. Of course, a vastly enhanced global trading network introduced new drugs to Indian medical systems (as well as in China) from the seventeenth century, just as they exponentially expanded the apothecaries' range of remedies in Britain and the Netherlands. Sarsaparilla, rhubarb, and, most spectacularly, cinchona and its febrifuges are such examples. While practitioners of Western medicine prescribed quinine pills, Indigenous medical practitioners in colonial India extensively used cinchona febrifuges not just as a fever cure, but also for dozens of ailments. Even Western medical practitioners prescribed quinine pills as general tonics in the nineteenth century in India, while disparate medical men in the bazaars dispensed quinine for all ailments.[63] The advantages of Western medicine were most visible in preventive medicine – sanitation and vaccination – and in advances in surgical or diagnostic techniques. The discovery of hormonal products such as insulin and vitamins enhanced the repertoire of commercial therapies.[64] Therefore, although the competition among drug traders and practitioners of Western or Indigenous medicine generated heated debate, they competed for the entire medical market and their products ranged across the epistemic and polemic boundaries of Western/Eastern medical systems.[65] This made legitimation by the government more relevant to them. Legislation promised validation for the relevant practitioners and manufacturers, and the government, being a purchaser of medicines for its hospitals, was a significantly influential customer. Therefore, the long struggle and negotiations for legislation and control of the drugs market and its corollaries, the training of dispensers and pharmacists, the intense debates on the potency and legitimate use of specific Indigenous drugs and medical therapies, and the publication of an Indian pharmacopeia (for Western therapies) all proved intense, fractious, and enduring. These battles were enacted in the public sphere and became part of the larger causes of scientific education, nationalist enterprise, and the promise of public health in modern India. It was only the drug legislations in the final years of British rule in India, of 1940 and 1944, that standardized the quality of medical therapies and standards of medical education enabled the new nation-state to plan for self-sufficiency in medical supplies. The final chapter of the book argues that the independent nation-state planned for and invested in biomedicine and institutions that facilitated its intensive use. It concludes that despite a political commitment to Indigenous medicine during the nationalist era, biomedicine gained momentum and eclipsed Indigenous medical systems in independent India. This book analyses these politics of making medicines in modern India.

1

The Colonial Medicine Chest

In the late nineteenth century, drugs, medicines, and potions filled the urban and mofussil markets and bazaars of India. Labelled bottles and jars of tinctures and powders were placed on the polished display shelves of the European shops in the 'white towns' of the metropolises. They were piled high, still in their packing boxes, freshly stamped from the docks in the more modest 'local' retailers. In even smaller shops or shacks in the native bazaars, medicines, herbs, spices, and mixtures spilled over from gunny sacks. Nor was it only the products themselves that were on display. Bold images of coloured bottles and carved medicine chests; virile men, fertile women, and healthy children who, having partaken of the required therapeutic substance, were filled with an enviable liveliness were visible daily in the press and across the city on leaflets, posters, and painted advertisements on walls both in English and the regional languages. The urban scape of modern India, in short, was saturated with a variety of medical remedies for sale.

This explosion of therapeutic commodities and the vast expansion in the Indian medical market occurred in the context of a burgeoning, somewhat ambivalently self-identifying, middle class in India. It reflected, more generally, a consumer culture that informed the public sphere in India at multiple levels. Medicines and therapeutic commodities, like other aspects of consumer culture, were in demand and very visible to the public; these comprised a range that included items of everyday use to objects of luxury. They also represented yet another site of the conflictual relationship between colonial modernity and emergent Indian selfhood.

This relationship has been studied in some depth. The colonial Indian emergent public sphere and a sense of nationhood among its literate communities were locked in between intense admiration and awe for Western institutions, values, and the material forms of the many institutions that these generated and a deep distrust of them. This was particularly true of feats of Western science/engineering. Therefore, the imposing Gothic architecture, piped water in cities, and the railways induced awe and wonder as well as deep, civilizational self-doubt and sustained mono-cultural revivalism within many sections of Indian society.[1] Simultaneously, it gradually introduced a sustained change in taste for consumer goods, some humble and others more luxurious. David Arnold has suggested that Indians appropriated, culturally, Western technology at various 'everyday' levels with the example of the extension of the use of bicycles and sewing machines that came to be objects of daily use in colonial India. The trope of 'appropriation' or cultural indigenisation, if you like, can be extended to items of everyday use that were the products of both technological sophistication and glossy packaging.[2]

Consumer culture in therapeutic goods in colonial India, therefore, was often ambivalent. Scholars have traced it from mimicry to self-fashioning of identity and nationalism.[3] As Karl Gerth has pointed out, in China as much as in India, it was not just consumption but also the boycott of foreign products that framed and politicised the market for branded and packaged commodities of everyday use.[4] It was not only at the site of machine-made Lancashire textiles that the battles for the Indian consumer self were manifest; these were represented and articulated in the public sphere and at the market place for therapeutic and cosmetic goods as much as clothes, carpets, and artefacts for the newly fashioned drawing rooms of the expanding middle classes from the nineteenth century onwards. From British-Indian households to the professional and commercial middle classes, India represented a buoyant market for consumer products of everyday use. In the mid-nineteenth century, these changing tastes were served by British and occasionally Continental imports. Later, the growth and subsequent segmentation among consumers of differing purchasing powers, as well as the political intervention of the Swadeshi/economic nationalism in public discourse, extended this market to the Indian traders, distributors, and eventually manufacturers.[5]

This expansion of the market for consumer goods was underwritten by the infrastructures of the colonial state. These included sustained tariff protections for British goods, an extended railway network throughout British and large parts of princely India, an all-India postal service that offered the opportunity to pay on delivery, and the establishment of retail stores in the mofussil and hill stations. Although therapeutic commodities can be classed as essential products, therapeutic commodities and ancillary cosmetic ones, such as toothpaste, body lotions, talcum powder, shaving brushes, and soap, etc., belonged to the category of branded consumer goods that were novel and desirable and available in a range of selections and through several modes of distribution in urban India.[6] Although every item of consumption, especially those understood as being produced by 'Western' technology, was also the site of political contestation, the variety and volume of items of consumption rose along with the burgeoning middle classes.[7]

The Colonial Medicine Chest

The initial extension of the prepared drugs market occurred through the use of the medicine chest. The medicine chest, of course, was not unique to colonial India. One of the most striking artefacts of the narratives of David Livingstone's quests for the source of the Nile deep into Africa in the mid-nineteenth century is his medicine chest.[8] Indeed, a 'medicine chest' of essential drugs and surgical materials was one of the most critical items of baggage for any colonial traveller to tropical worlds in the nineteenth century. Not just isolated explorers. Missionaries, officials in remote outposts, and housewives who joined their husbands in less isolated but nonetheless provincial stations by the mid-nineteenth century packed a medicine chest for their journey to the East.

As historians have amply demonstrated, representations of tropical landscapes changed from being wondrous, abundant, and rich with a multitude of mineral and botanical treasures to ones that were darker and more threatening from the sixteenth to the eighteenth centuries.[9] Naturally enough, these perceptions followed changing narratives of what comprised the 'tropics' itself. Tropical terrors included malaria, a multitude of fevers, sleeping sickness, and, of course, cholera, dreaded the most for the swift and painful death. Cholera became a quintessential tropical disease and Europeans located its 'home' in the malignant swamps of lower Bengal. The fear – sheer, physical horror – of entering the interior of the tropics and encountering sudden and fatal illness remained with Europeans long after they had established empires and identified tropical landscapes not just in the New World or in Asia, but in most places beyond Europe.[10] The need for medicine chests remained as well; they changed in shape, size, and content but remained essential for travel beyond the Suez Canal until the commencement of the Second World War.

Although drugs of botanical and mineral origins were traded in the premodern world, early modern global trade networks expanded the sheer numbers of drugs available to apothecaries in the Western world.[11] The establishment of botanical gardens and experimental replanting and transfer of plant material throughout the world, and particularly within the British Empire, further extended the repertoire of therapeutic drugs for daily use in industrialised nations.[12] By the nineteenth century, the international trade in raw and crude botanical drugs had widened to a global network of exchange and experimentation with planting botanical products, most used in therapeutic products. At the site of distribution of these in the form of finished products, the apothecaries, the newer profession of 'chemists and druggists', and physicians struggled to define their specific roles and limit the functions of the relatively low skilled practitioners such as midwives and 'wise women' of an earlier era. The establishment of the Pharmaceutical Society of Britain in 1851 professionalised the 'chemists and druggists' occupation, although the power struggle among different branches of the medical profession that interacted directly with patients and were involved with dispensing and prescribing drugs and medicines continued late into the nineteenth century.[13] In Scotland, for instance, general physicians continued to supplement their incomes with dispensing medicines themselves to their patients.

Along with the expansion in the number of therapeutic drugs, innovations in manufacturing and marketing, such as tablets rather than old-style powders and branded and proprietary therapeutic products that were relatively easy to store and transport facilitated the expansion of pharmaceutical products.[14] The Burroughs Wellcome &Co.'s (B.W.&Co.) compressed tabloids and medicine chests are a celebrated example. The medicine chests and their contents represented not just the convenience of having prepared medical remedies at hand, but they were also solicitously marketed as agents of modern medicine and progress in the outposts of the British Empire.[15] Although medicine chests were commonly used by ship surgeons from the seventeenth century, in the

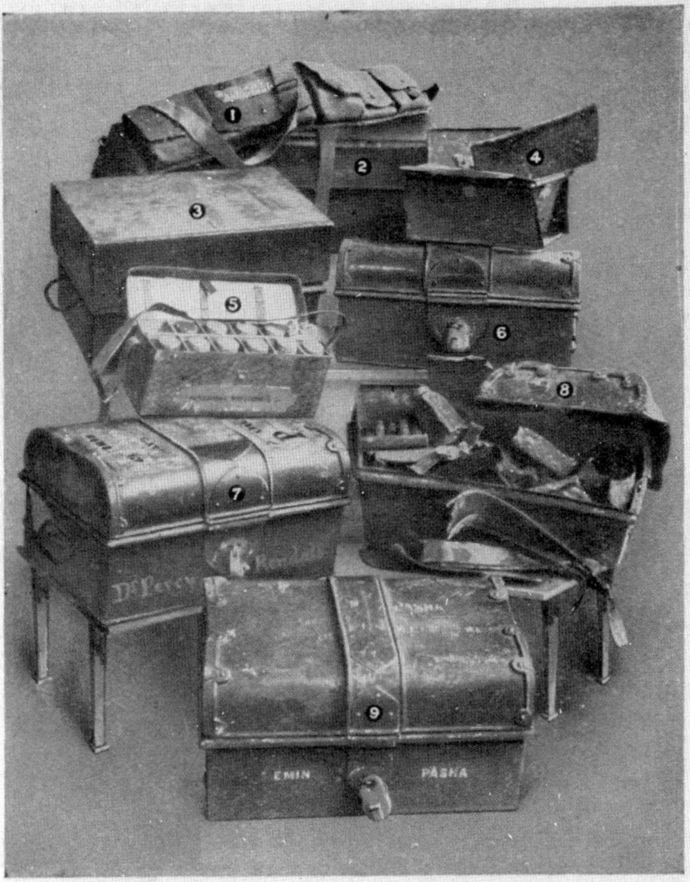

RELIC 'TABLOID' MEDICINE CASES—AFRICA

1—Medicine Belt carried by Capt. Stairs throughout his Katanga Expedition. 2—The famous "Rear-Guard" Medicine Chest used during Sir H. M. Stanley's travels. 3—Extricated from the ruins after the Bandawe Mission House had been demolished by lightning; the contents that escaped damage were used for more than ten years afterwards. 4—Once the property of E. G. Glave. Supplied for a journey made concerning the great slave question of Central Africa. This Case was afterwards damaged in the Brussels Exhibition Fire, 1910. 5—Carried by Capt. Thomas Stevens on the Expedition in East Africa to find Stanley. 6—Chest carried by Sir H. M. Stanley during the Emin Pasha Relief and other Expeditions. 7—Formerly the property of Dr. Percy Rendall, Principal Medical Officer, British Central Africa Administration. 8—Case carried by Frank Muxworthy, the famous African Caravan Leader, on three journeys through Uganda. 9—The last Medicine Chest supplied to Emin Pasha. This Chest was also damaged in the Brussels Exhibition Fire, 1910.

Figure 1.1 Tabloid Medicine Chest Africa

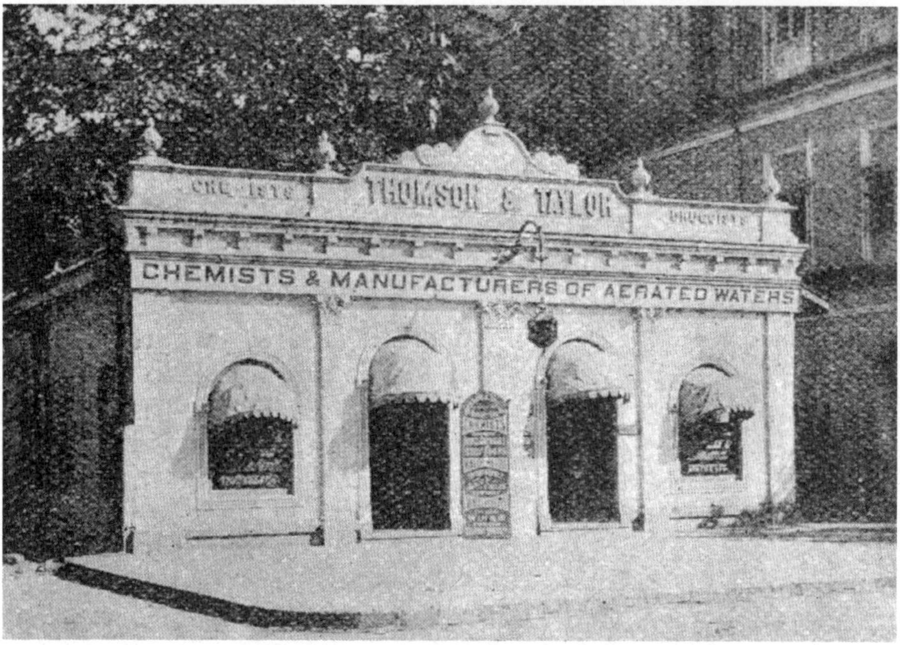

Figure 1.2 Thomson & Taylor's pharmacy, exterior, *Chemist and Druggist*, 19 April 1902

late nineteenth century these were used regularly by non-medical travellers or settlers.

The colonial medicine chests are, therefore, both material artefacts that allow us to examine the diverse contents of the druggists' therapies temporally as well as a metaphor for the pharmaceutalisation of colonial societies. Pharmaceutalisation is a term largely used by sociologists and anthropologists to refer to a set of diagnoses that medical authority determines to require clinical intervention in the contemporary age. But if we can broaden the usage of the term to include the extension of the marketing of medical therapies to colonial subjects in the late nineteenth century, pharmaceutalisation raises interesting questions for the colonial historian.

The medicine chests served to popularise the dispensing of therapeutic remedies from the industrialised nations to the Atlantic and the tropical worlds wherever emigrants, settlers, or colonial officials travelled.[16] For these medicine chests (available in different sizes according to one's convenience and means) and the compressed boxes of powders, bottles of liquid tinctures, and antiseptic surgical material within them represented the scientific and miraculous prowess of Western medicine to the subjugated civilisations in Africa, the Pacific Islands, or within their older Asian rivals. The medicine chests facilitated wider marketing of therapeutic products across the British Empire. Like many other British commodities, the market for therapeutic products was complex, crowded, and contested terrain, but at the same time offered a plenitude of opportunity for expansion. This expansion occurred in the context of innovative means of marketing and distribution and in the shadow of the constant threat of alternative therapies available in a very heterogeneous market.

The Medical Market in Colonial India

Historians have generally understood this expansion of packaged therapeutic commodities through the analyses of the cultures of consumption in colonial societies and through the analytical category of 'colonial modernity', which is generally placed in conflict with the premodern or the pre-colonial. And while the category of colonial modernity is conflictual and fragmented, it nonetheless encapsulates the vast changes and disjuncture that were experienced by colonised peoples in the European colonial empires. In colonial India, these included changes in agrarian policy and relations, the impoverishment of large sections of peasantry over the nineteenth century, and, consequently, famine and depopulation in rural areas as well as the simultaneous expansion of a Western-educated, professional urban middle class. The emergent self-identifying middle classes in India at the turn of the nineteenth century were ambivalent and fragmentary but defined themselves through consumption.[17] The rise in the use of consumer goods, whether everyday goods such as liquors, chocolate, health tonics, or cutlery; or luxury items like watches, cameras, pianos, and motor cars, is presumed on the mostly urban elite within colonial south Asia. It is they who made the best use of Western institutions such as universities, law courts, and hospitals and who, through an explosion in vernacular and English language presses, formed and participated in the public sphere. They were employed as doctors, lawyers, civil servants, or as absentee landlords through the new rules of agrarian property and were able to grasp the opportunities provided by the colonial state to establish themselves as the most vocal and articulate members of Indian society.

However, if we can move beyond understanding pharmaceutalization in colonial India from the perspective of the culture/s of consumption and focus on the distribution of commodities; in this case, therapeutic commodities, it opens other possibilities of looking at the fast expansion of the medical market in south and Southeast Asia. For instance, we can ask how and to what extent the colonial states were implicated in the patronage of therapeutic goods. And this question is significant, for apart from government hospitals, dispensaries and laboratories formed a substantial part of the medical infrastructure available in South Asia. An examination of the infrastructure building by the colonial states – through the extension of railways, the ubiquitous and reliable postal and telegraph services, and the shipping lines – will help us to view the extension of the medical market. We can also explore the networks and connections between medical men, whether official or non-official practitioners, who were educated in Britain and the pharmaceutical companies based in their home country.

In the early nineteenth century, metropolitan drug companies liaised with the India Office in London and received large contracts for the supply of drugs and surgical products directly to the East India Company.[18] This continued after the dissolution of the EIC in 1858, and bulk orders were booked from the office of the Secretary of State for India. These were used principally in army hospitals. As the colonial state consolidated its regime, it established government hospitals with IMS officials on special civilian duties in charge – these too acquired all drugs and therapeutic materials from the India Office. As the hospital and dispensary system within the Western medicine system expanded to include smaller, charitable institutions in the provincial districts and the princely states encouraged by the government and supported by Indian philanthropy, the military medical establishment supplied therapeutic products to these institutions. This was done through five Government Medical Stores (GMS); one in each of the Madras, Bengal, Bombay, the north-western provinces, and the fifth in Burma.

Yet these hospitals and dispensaries served little more than a fraction of the population. In 1916, in an impassioned debate on government support for Indigenous medical institutions in the Legislative Council of India, one member pointed out the inadequacy of government-aided dispensaries and hospitals: 'There are 4,400 dispensaries all over British India treating about 38 million patients … there are but five medical colleges with about 1,700 students and 28 medical schools with about 4,200 pupils for all India'.[19] People bought therapeutic remedies from a disparate medley of medical practitioners. These ranged from the very expensive private consultations offered by the Indian Medical Service officers, which were used chiefly by the British and the elite Indians, to trained Indian doctors from the new Western medical colleges, and others who had attended a year or two of medical college but had not achieved a full degree.[20] When provincial governments implemented the Medical Registration Acts (1912–14), which were an attempt to curb the expansion of private medical colleges, especially in the presidency capitals of Calcutta, Madras, and Bombay, it was not only the private practitioners of 'Western' medicine who objected. District officials in the mofussils also voiced their reservations, pointing out that the graduates (or even non-graduates) from the private medical colleges provided a vital service, and their only rivals in the district towns or rural areas were the Indigenous practitioners whose medical knowledge or training could be even more suspect. As a district collector in north Bengal pointed out, 'It is desirable that the public should know what they are paying for, but until medical men are a good deal more common than they are at present the mofussil public will, … be glad to pay for what they can get without enquiring too closely into its quality'.[21] Other medical practitioners included homeopaths, vaidyas (also known as baidya or kaviraj in Bengal), and hakims who learnt their skills traditionally from practising medical men, as well as those who obtained diplomas from the new colleges in Ayurveda and Unani medicine.[22] Since there was no legislation to restrain anyone from practising medicine, spice sellers, itinerant peddlers, and most pharmacists also offered medical consultations along with their therapeutic products.

Disparate remedies and eclectic practitioners flourished in this environment. Qualified Western medical practitioners prescribed Ayurvedic remedies for a host of illnesses. Ayurvedas offered injectable medication, traditional *haad vaids* (bone-setters) performed surgeries and prescribed a diverse range of medicines. Homeopathy, unipathy, hydropathy, naturopathy, electropathy, every medical caprice or innovation found accommodation and a market in colonial India. To cater to this diverse medical culture, transnational drug companies devised methods that would extend their markets far beyond their swanky retail outlets in the metropolitan cities. This is where we come back to the colonial's medical chest: they used the iconic 'tropical medical chests' to persuade the medical consumers in the provincial districts, remote hill stations, and outposts of the empire to buy their products. The contents of the medical chest became ever more innovative at the turn of the century. It is well known that B.W.& Co. manufactured the first tropical medical chests that were used by explorers including David Livingstone, in Africa. B.W.& Co was also the first to manufacture compressed tablets, branding them tabloids that distinguished them from the competitors who followed their example.[23] The designs, weight, and shape of the medicine chests acquired diversity. There were large, heavy boxes that would be carried by African labourers over long distances and could be fitted with a selection of tabloids, powders, bandages, and instruments to meet any eventuality in the unknown tropical territory. These were different from the Indian medical chests, which were much smaller and intended for everyday domestic use, and could be replenished conveniently. Bruce and Company's medical chest for India, for instance, listed around sixty-three products in 1843, including the Cholera Pill, surgical needle and thread, and the intriguingly named Blue Pill and Dinner Pill, as well as more everyday remedies such as Dover's powder, opium, laudanum, and sulphate of quinine.[24] But the accompanying manual assured prospective customers that 'the above comprises the contents of the largest Chest that is made; smaller ones do not contain the whole of them, only the *most useful*, according to the number of bottles and price of the chest'.[25] In 1878, James White, formerly civil surgeon of Rangoon, recommended forty-three essential drugs including quinine, cholera pills, and the ubiquitous blue pills for any medicine chest for merchants' ships without a surgeon.[26] The manufacturing chemists of London, Godfrey and Cook's, recommended only around thirty articles in their '*The A.B.C. of Domestic Medicine, or Companion to the Medicine Chest, for the Use of Travellers and Families at a Distance from Medical Assistance*' around a decade later.[27] The isolation of their active principles from many botanical products enabled the compression of the bulk of medicines easily. When Spencer Thomson, MD, LRCS (Edinburgh) wrote an introduction to Messrs Richardson and Company of Leicester's Colonists Medical Chest in 1874, he could claim that:

> Within the last few years, the improved preparations of drugs, and the power of administering many of their active principles free from extraneous matter, has greatly facilitated their preparations in the form of pills, and the various methods of coating these have rendered them not only more agreeable to take, but more easy to keep them in preservation. Hence … Pill Chest … of Messrs Richardson and Co of Leicester, has been designed and constructed by them so as to contain, in the compact form of pills, such a selection of medicines as would be most likely to meet immediate wants, more especially in places far distant from the usual conveniences of settled society. Moreover, the medicines, though few in no, are so selected as to be capable, under guidance … to meet very varied indications, … the pills being cut, into halves or quarters, or as in or two instances, broken down altogether.[28]

Therefore, different sizes of medicine chests with divergent therapies were also marketed to specific consumer groups. In 1909, B.W. & Co. was advertising its India medicine chest to missionaries:

> Most missionaries, even if not qualified physicians, have had a course of medical training, and therefore possess a practical knowledge of common remedies, and are in a position to administer them ….
>
> All such must have noted the variability which exists in the ordinary medicines on the market, and the difficulty which is sometimes experienced in obtaining products which are reliable … This difficulty is at once overcome by using BW and Co products, which contain only the finest drugs, and are exceptional in therapeutic activity, purity, uniformity and reliability … Tabloid and Soloid products are particularly suitable for missionary use; … easily carried … keep well in every climate.[29]

A large educated middle class dominated the consumption cultures of principal cities in colonial India. These included not only the presidency capitals of Bombay, Calcutta, and Madras but also large provincial towns such as Delhi, Benares, Allahabad, Lahore, Patna, Bangalore, Poona, and Cochin. Large towns flourished in the hill stations where most of British-Indian officialdom lived and worked for more than half the year, the largest of these were

Simla, Darjeeling, and Ootacamund. The administrative capitals of prosperous princely states such as Hyderabad, Baroda, and Travancore also grew in size and population in the late nineteenth century. A lively urban culture developed in colonial India the cities and towns were the locations of the successes of the colonial economy and polity; of large British, Anglo-Indian, and educated Indians as well as migrant labourers, servants, traders, shopkeepers, and small and large manufacturers.

The emergence of the medical consumer in colonial India, therefore, is problematic for disparate cultures of medicine production as well as marketing. The consumers were mostly urban or semi-urban, socially diverse but broadly belonging to the lower-middle to middle classes. The making of a modern middle class in India was a fragmented and ambivalent process, but these urban and semi-urban centres, therapeutics, and medicine assumed not just political but also commercial overtones. In eighteenth-century India, both Western and Indigenous medical systems such as Ayurveda and Unani depended, for the most part, on herbs and their extracts, minerals and their compounds, and extracts of animal matter (like various apothecaries in England) for their therapies. The East India Company surgeons also depended greatly on the local markets for their therapies, and their medical items included, heterogeneously, hundreds of botanical and mineral products locally available from native dispensers who were often also spice merchants. These were known as 'bazaar medicines'.[30] Throughout the eighteenth and early nineteenth century, bazaar medicines, vaguely defined, constituted a significant but declining proportion of the EEIC's total expenditure on therapeutics. These supplemented, but never replaced, the total quantity of drugs used by government medical institutions in the nineteenth century. The trade in therapeutic products was differentiated according to both scale and production; at one end were the 'European' drug houses that catered to the British-Indian community and to the aristocratic and the affluent; at the other were the drug sellers in local bazaars who sold crude drugs as well as locally made generic medicines. Within this wide spectrum were the importers, traders, manufacturers of Indigenous and allopathic remedies, and retailers and distributors who participated in the vast sub-Continental drugs market.

'European' Drug Houses: Expanding the Medical Market

By far the largest and most lucrative share of the drugs trade was initially monopolized by the large British-owned retailers who imported drugs from Britain and manufactured a few basic drugs and cosmetics from local materials or from imported bulk drugs. From the mid-nineteenth century when the colonial state extended its patronage and encouraged the establishment of therapeutic institutions on the Western model such as hospitals and charitable dispensaries, these institutions variously used drugs procured from England. In the late nineteenth century, the flow of drugs represented a classically metropolis-colony relationship. Britain imported a huge number of crude drugs from India; these were processed in some form and exported back to the colony. A large proportion of these drugs were bought by the army in India for the use of its troops in army hospitals. The Indian army also extensively purchased all kinds of pharmaceutical preparations and proprietary medicines from abroad. Since the expansion of the hospital system in colonial India was first undertaken and then overseen by military administration, the supply of medicines to them was undertaken by the medical department of the colonial government. Therefore, the government was the biggest purchaser of Western therapeutic products at the turn of the century. The five GMSs, in Calcutta, Bombay, Madras, Lahore, and Rangoon, also purchased raw drugs and chemicals in the bazaars, processed them in their workshops, and stored them in their warehouses, which were called 'factories'.

The military in British India was, therefore, both a manufacturer and supplier of drugs to the government-aided hospitals and dispensaries. Although they were supposedly sold at discounted rates to civil institutions, the Medical Store Department (MSD) profited from being the sole supplier. The army did not record the exact value of the profits made from sales to civilian institutions; nevertheless, the first annual report in 1909 pointed out that if these sales were discontinued, a heavy burden would be thrown on the military budget'.[31] Apart from obtaining a few drugs and processing them locally, in the late nineteenth century, the MSD's regional offices preferred to patronise firms from England. Large manufacturing firms in England had agents in Bombay or Calcutta who negotiated contracts with the government on their behalf.[32]

Outside of government-aided institutions, the private market flourished. In the early twentieth century, urban areas in British India became the sites of competition for the distribution and sale of numerous medicines, usually imported from Britain, Germany, the USA, and even Japan. This also facilitated the entry and presence of several pharmaceutical multinational companies (MNCS) and the Indian pharmaceutical market became a lucrative area for foreign companies. Some of the major companies involved in exporting pharmaceutical products to India included B.W.& Co. and Burgoyne and Burbidges (UK), Parke, Davis and Co., (USA), McKesson and Robbins, Bayer, and Glaxo. This consumer market in therapeutic products refers not only to drugs, but also to a range of cosmetic and consumer products such as aerated water, hair oil, creams and ointments, toothpaste, aphrodisiacs, and tonics for invalids of all ages. The drugs themselves included patented medicines as well as generic 'cholera' pills, 'fever pills', 'stomach pills', and innumerable varieties of aphrodisiacs. The development and dissemination of nutrition research in the inter-war years subsequently prompted the demand for a rise in vitamin products, particularly when certain strands of thought within Indian nationalism advocated for the development of strong, virile, muscular Indian bodies to counter the supposedly stronger British.

In the late nineteenth century, the bulk of the drugs was sold by British or European firms that imported drugs. These firms were based in the colonial metropolises of Calcutta, Bombay, and Madras. They catered mostly to the European (White, mostly British) clientele both in the cities and in the hill stations, district headquarters, industrial enclaves, and commercial hubs where the European population of India resided. The largest of the British-owned firms were Treacher and Co. (Bombay and Poona), Frank, Ross and Co. (Calcutta), Kemp and Co. (Bombay), Messrs Phillip and Co. (Bombay), Bathgate and Co. (Calcutta), Martin and Harris (Calcutta), Symes and Co. (Simla and Umballa), and W.E. Smith and Sons (Madras). These large companies sold pharmaceuticals in retail, but this was only part of their widespread business concerns. They also procured and sold wholesale drugs for large British-owned companies in India, including the several rail and tea companies and collieries that needed to distribute basic drugs such as compounds of cinchona, for example, on a large scale to their workers, or to the native states that built therapeutic institutions for the public, such as Baroda, Travancore, and Hyderabad.[33] As mentioned before, pharmaceutical companies in Britain and Germany also had their own agents who negotiated contracts on their behalf with the large wholesale firms, with one agent often working for two or even three firms simultaneously. So, there was a complex hierarchy of manufacturers' agents, wholesalers, retailers, and bazaar pharmacists operating in the Indian market at this time.

In the nineteenth century, the largest demand for imported drugs, cosmetics, and related goods was from British/European settlements in India. Europeans resident in India patronised 'European' (British-owned) establishments to supply them with many necessities of what they considered to be a comfortable and 'civilized' life. They depended on metropolitan imports for many articles of daily use – umbrellas, cutlery, photographic equipment, perfumes, cosmetics; sewing machines and gramophones – as well as preserved fruits; medicated wines; brandies and spirits; tobacco; canned meats, especially ham; cocoa; chocolate; and invariably, bottles of patent medicines, powders, and medicine chests. Apart from the metropolitan centres at Bombay and Calcutta, European importers of pharmaceuticals and other cosmetic goods first established themselves near large cantonment towns such as Poona, Ambala, Meerut, Kanpur, and Secunderabad; also in hill stations at Simla, Darjeeling, and Ootacamund. In the 1880s, there were a few large British-owned firms that competed to market their goods to retailers and directly to consumers all over British India and in the native states. They bought most of their supplies from exporters, who all had 'agents' who often handled the businesses of several manufacturers and exporters from Britain simultaneously. They were, in effect, large wholesalers who based themselves in the colonial port towns. In his caricature of the 'types' of Europeans in India, a contemporary observed the 'European Merchant' as a gentleman trader ensconced in a metropolitan port, 'You seldom find the "Gentleman" Merchant inland … Of course, at Bombay, Calcutta, Madras and Kurrachee he is in force, a power to be reckoned with. He chiefly exports crude country produce … while he may import spirits, Manchester stuffs, Sheffield cutlery'.[34]

These European importers and their British employees, like other 'non-official' British residents in India, were a part of the 'boxwallah' community.[35] Like most British traders in colonial India, they engaged in a varied trade that included importing and manufacturing of wholesale and retail goods.[36] They produced a variety of goods themselves including aerated water, which was in great demand among Europeans in India and guaranteed profits for all producers. It was also relatively easy to produce, and, therefore, almost all European pharmacies in India manufactured and marketed aerated water on their own premises.[37] European firms also procured contracts for the supply of aerated water to government institutions including the Governor General's establishment. Here they often competed with the Indian army itself and resented what they thought was an unfair competition:

> The aerated water trade is being much cut into by the regimental messes, who are large consumers. They buy a machine, manufacture their own waters, and sell them to customers at greatly reduced prices. A petition has gone up to the Viceroy from the tradespeople, protesting against the soldiers competing with them in this way.[38]

Another consumer product that found a large, ready-made market was soaps. The history of the marketing of soaps in tropical colonies has been analysed by historians who have pointed out that it was linked inextricably to the civilizing mission in Africa.[39] Indeed it was, and as the triumphant advertisements of the Pears soap demonstrate, commerce, conquest, conversion, and the civilizing mission were close partners in the tropical colonies. In India, the market for soaps was slightly different at this time; it was sold largely to European residents through British retailers. Although soap was one of the first small industries to be developed in India and was produced by several Indian manufacturers in the late nineteenth century, the demand for British soap remained constant and even increased in twentieth-century India; 'In the past soap trade has been almost exclusively in British hands … not only is the volume of this trade increasing, but that the British imports represent each year a greater proportion of the total … an example of what may be achieved by enterprise and strict attention to the requirements of the Indian market'.[40]

However, the main business of the British importing firms was procuring and selling a huge number of imported generic, patent, and proprietary medicines; in time, they manufactured their own patent medicines and mixtures. The expansion of the bureaucracy and military establishments of the Raj in the post-1858 period, therefore, fostered a community of British consumers of European medical and allied goods.

This marketing of therapeutic consumer items to the British residents in India could begin before their first voyage. Indeed, prospective travellers, including civil servants, visitors, and missionaries who expected to live away from the urban centres were advised to purchase a 'medicine chest' from any reputed manufacturer in Britain before embarking on the journey.[41] The British trade journal *The Chemist and Druggist* urged young and ambitious pharmacists among its readers in Britain to look for opportunities in India and establish a business in the "newly-opened out" territories of the Deccan, or the hill stations that were rapidly expanding in this period. These pharmacies provided for Europeans as well as aristocratic Indians; most of their products were too expensive for the Indian pockets, even those of the middle and professional classes. They employed British and Eurasian assistants but a great part of the manual work of grinding and mixing the powders and tinctures was done by Indian assistants. In the absence of either a food and drugs law or a self-governing body of pharmacists, the quality of the goods varied; therefore, each prominent retail store depended on its own name brand for marketing its products. In many cantonment towns and hill stations, these stores were a part of the commercial landscape. The Bombay-based Treacher and Company had achieved virtually a monopoly over European pharmaceutical products in Poona, a cantonment town near Bombay. So much so, they printed a guidebook for visitors to Poona in 1876; their outlet was located on Arsenal Road, also known informally as the Treacher Road.[42] Similarly, the large shop and display window of Frank, Ross and Company dominated the Commercial Row in the hill station of Darjeeling in Bengal. In Kanpur, a manufacturing town originally specialising in saddlery and boots for the Company's army, a growing number of industrial units established through British capital employed a significant number of Europeans in managerial positions.[43] It boasted of several European drug houses that supplied the British-Indian community.[44]

While the large importers lived in the coastal metropolises, the 'tradesman', located a few rungs below in British society, were numerous in the metropolises, and each district town had at least one or two.[45] The hill stations of British India such as Simla, Darjeeling, and Ootacamund, where the central and provincial governments retreated for half the year with their clerical and menial staff, and where many British families resided permanently, also accommodated large

'European pharmacies' that catered to the affluent retail trade as well as distributed their products to tradesmen with a more modest clientele.

> Prescriptions are many and varied, from the humble calomel powder to the most complicated mixture which the medical mind may formulate. From all parts of the world they have originated- Harley Street, Paris, New York, Naples, Cairo, Athens, Berlin: all have their representatives ... He may be called upon to answer the questions and supply the demands of his Excellency or even those of the humble native shopman.[46]

The European traders in Bombay, Madras, Rangoon, and Calcutta engaged directly with suppliers from Britain as well as with their agents. Mr Charles W. White, for instance, represented Burgoyne, Burbidges and Co., A.F. Pears, and B.W.& Co. in India. While he was a larger-than-life figure, well known to all British and several Indian wholesalers, he was only one of several. As the Indian correspondent of *Chemist and Druggist* pointed out in 1899, 'Mr White is so well known and popular, that his regular visits are appreciated. Messrs Baiss Bros. And Co. have also a representative about to do India; whilst Messrs Evans, Lescher, and Webb and Lynch and Co. have permanent resident agencies but recently established'.[47]

These 'drug houses' used English dailies and periodicals as well as printed catalogues and circulars posted by mail order to reach their audience. Apart from the retail units and the large government contracts, (where they depended upon personal connections), they marketed their goods and those of the other companies through advertisements in newspapers, periodicals, and in the few medical journals. Both the English and the Indian newspapers contained large advertisements by leading druggists as well as manufacturers. The European companies targeted the British-Indian consumers through the leading Anglo-Indian dailies such as the *Pioneer Mail* (Allahabad), *Civil and Military Gazette* (Lahore), as well as *The Times of India* (Bombay) and the *Statesman* (Calcutta), but they also addressed specialized periodicals such as the *Bombay Guardian*, a missionary periodical where Kemp and Co., for instance, regularly advertised their numerous products: 'Special Terms to Missionaries and Charitable Institutions' to evangelists who lived and travelled in remote districts and delivered 'drug, chemicals, surgical instruments, patent medicines, proprietary articles' by post.[48]

The elite metropolitan retailers used their status as suppliers to highly placed officials to further their own image as dealers in exclusive and special goods. W.E. Smith of Madras, for instance, appealed to be nominated as 'Chemists to H.R.H. Prince of Wales' in 1906 because their agency had supplied a few medical supplies to the royal's entourage during his recent tour to Madras.[49]

The distributors also directly canvassed medical professionals, both official and non-official. Until the agitation for economic nationalism (Swadeshi movement) in 1905, the European companies had almost a monopoly over supplying government contracts as well as British companies, such as collieries, railways, and plantations in India.

Another way of advertising their products and canvassing for trade was to attend or send their wares to industrial exhibitions. Especially after the Empire Exhibition in London, industrial exhibitions provided both spectacle and functionality to exporting and importing firms as well as manufacturing pharmacies in India. The first was held in Calcutta in 1884; later, nationalists and princely states held industrial exhibitions of their own, showcasing Swadeshi manufacture. The exhibitions represented ways to display products as well as to do business directly with medical professionals. In the Calcutta exhibition of 1884, well-known British manufacturers such as Ferris and Co., of Bristol; Evans, Sons and Co. of Liverpool; Evans, Lescher and Webb, of London; Hewlett and Son, of London; Burgoyne, Burbidges and Co.; the Maltine Manufacturing Company Ltd.; Arnold and Sons, of London; and B.W.& Co. all displayed their special products, packaging, and catalogues to prospective importers. Here there was a 'Foreign Court' that gave space to 'homeopathic medicines exhibited by Dr William Schwabe, of Leipzig; essences by Gustave Boehm, of Offenbach-am-Main and London; and in a wooden case … corks of several sizes and of excellent quality by A. Dauphin, of Stuttgart' as well as an 'Australian court' where the visitor could find 'exhibits of drugs, chemicals, soaps, extracts, etc. from the firm of Messrs Felton, Grimwade and Co, of Melbourne, and Mr J. Bosisto, of the same place'.[50]

Here, apart from large British manufacturers such as Treacher's, Stanistreet, Smith and Co.; Bathgate and Co.; David Waldie and Co.; etc., small-scale Indian manufacturers of tinctures, pills, and homeopathic medicines from Calcutta such as Mitra and Co., Tincoury Nandan, and Ghon and Son also took this opportunity to exhibit their oils, pills, and locally made instruments.[51]

The large importers in India also displayed favoured products, particularly from Britain. B.W.& Co., for instance, had to carefully proportion the number of its products and space that rival importers Bathgate and Co. and Smith, Stanistreet and Co. of Calcutta could each display at an industrial exhibition:

> This firm were [Bathgate and Co] the first to take up our goods in Calcutta and have pushed and advertised them considerably at their own expense.
>
> S.S. and Co are very good people but should not have any advantage over Bathgate at the Exhibition.
>
> Would recommend that you with Bathgate and Co and propose to send them some of our goods and exhibits with their own. Unless you do this they will have a grievance against us for they have done a good deal to introduce our goods and the houses are very jealous of S.S. and Co.[52]

At this period, the distributors of 'British-made' imported pharmaceutical products enjoyed unrivalled status and an almost mystical reputation for 'quality', as did any other consumer product that was imported, especially from the metropolis.[53] In 1882, a representative of the Fellows Medical Marketing & Manufacturing Co. of Sydney travelled to Bombay and wrote to Henry Wellcome that he fully expected to advance B.W.& Co.'s business in 'India, Burmah, and Thailand'.[54] He visited prominent drug retailers in Bombay who, he claimed, 'boast of importing everything from London or England (as the people here are strongly English) and their customers think nothing can be good unless it comes from England'.[55] Therefore the privilege of displaying well-known British names was treasured by distributors in India. The British manufacturing firms provided their own labels with space for the importer and distributors in India to place their own firms' names and addresses, providing for the advertisement of both the manufacturer and the wholesaler.

Once the presidency capital markets were saturated in the late nineteenth century, British importers and their travelling agents branched out to district towns and the regional cantonment towns and hill stations that housed substantial numbers of British residents.[56] Their extensive print advertisements and regular 'circulars' and letters to district civil surgeons (who enjoyed the

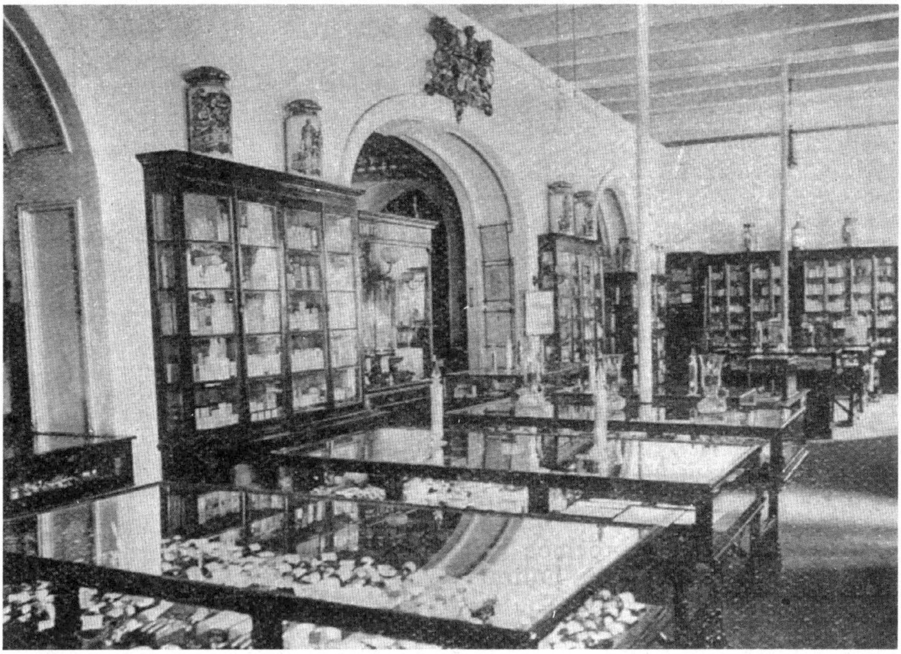

Figure 1.3 Inside the main retail store of Smith, Stanistreet and Company, Calcutta

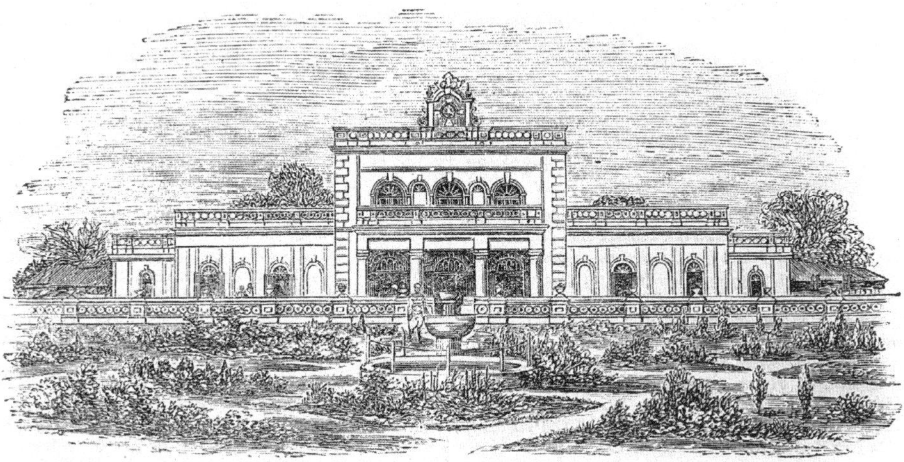

Figure 1.4 Lazarus and Company, Benares

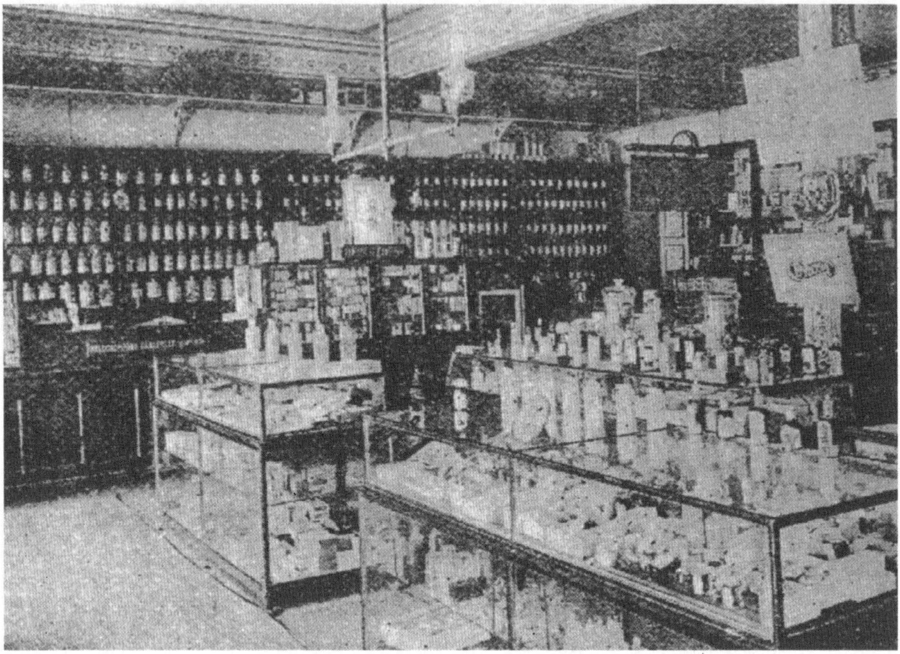

Figure 1.5 Interior of Thomson & Taylor, *Chemist and Druggist*, Bombay

privilege of private practice and was consulted by the British and the local Indian elite) and other privately practising physicians, British, or Anglo-Indian general stores that stored some therapeutic products, and charitable medical institutions such as missionary hospitals generated a large mail-order clientele. And in fact, in the colonial mofussil, all British residents and most Anglo-Indians shopped regularly from advertisements through the mail-order post; a contemporary observer compared the size of retailers' catalogues and price lists to the voluminous '*Field*'.[57] British residents who were away from the metropolitan cities relied heavily on the mail-order catalogues and the VPP (value payable post) postal system for their luxury and therapeutic items.[58]

Most British importing firms provided catalogues gratis by post on request and offered to send orders payable on delivery; this system was even more favoured when in 1904, the Government of India eliminated the payment of duty on the import of trade brochures and catalogues.[59] By the inter-war years, the VPP mail-order catalogue and the VPP system was entrenched. When the

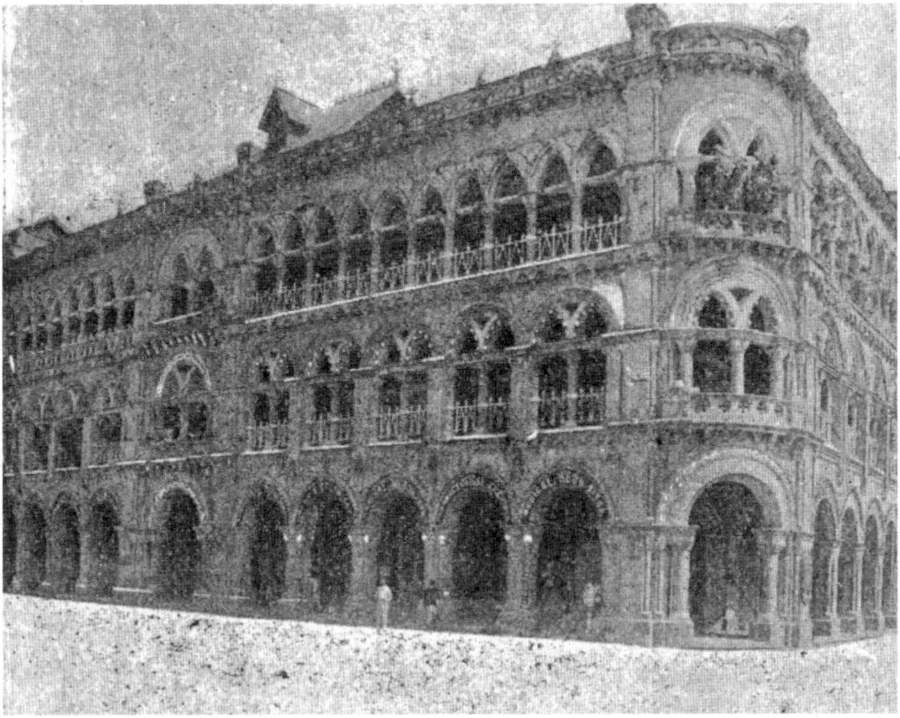

Figure 1.6 Kemp and Co., main premises, Bombay

Trade Commissioner of India and Ceylon urged British firms to compete with German and Japanese drug exporters by expanding their market, establishing stock depots in Bombay and Calcutta, and employing Indian travelling salesmen, he advised that 'The business can be worked comparatively easily and safely, and a large mail-order trade could be developed, utilising the admirable VPP system of the Indian Post Office'.[60]

Conclusion: New Markets in British India

At the turn of the century, India (along with southern Africa, the British Caribbean, Ceylon, and Australia) was a developing market for drugs and therapeutic products manufactured in Great Britain.[61] There are no reliable records for the total amount of manufacture and trading in drugs and pharmaceuticals in British India at this time. But apart from various anecdotal sources, a perusal of the number of companies that paid custom duty for the import of 'spirituous material', most of them for use in tinctures and drugs, provides us with several dozen exporters from England, France, Germany, and America.[62]

Transnational firms and their agents used new marketing strategies such as free samples and personal visits to physicians to ensure that their products remained visible and prescribed. This was most evident in the case of B.W.& Co., which fostered similar marketing strategies in Britain.[63] For instance, B.W.& Co. advised its main agent in India to arrange to send regular boxes of free samples of their products to all doctors in India and Ceylon:

> I think that the most effectual way to keep our goods before the Doctors in India is to send each one of them every two or three months a sample parcel … by all means send fair supplies of the article in question and to Bombay Calcutta Madras Colombo and also to our customers in the smaller towns in proportion and give code words by means of which additional quantities can be ordered by telegraph.[64]

B.W. & Co. provided special discounts to individual distributors in the major metropolises of Bombay, Calcutta, and Madras and also provided extra 'unique' discounts for their importers that distributed their products. Although the London firms used British-owned importer firms in the Indian subcontinent, keener exporters like B.W. & Co. did not allow their distributors to follow the usual norm of working for several British manufacturing firms simultaneously. By 1903, B.W. &Co. had access to orders from the Amir of Afghanistan and the firm sent instructions to their agent, 'We want to secure orders for our products from the Amir's Govt and also to keep any competing firms quite out of that market.[65]

The correspondences of B.W. & Co. show that in the 1880s, a network of international agents based in Bombay, Calcutta, Cape Town, and Melbourne represented an expansion area for emerging markets. The metropolitan sales agents dealt with the importing drugs firms in colonial cities; these, in turn, employed a string of touring salesmen who travelled to the provinces and mofussil districts, offering discounted contracts to wholesalers and large retailers. The wholesalers, in turn, employed salesmen who delivered sales literature offering the latest products to individual medical practitioners.

Therefore, besides the bulk government contracts, transnational firms like B.W. & Co. expanded their business by directly approaching provincial medical practitioners and their patients. Since medical practice was not regulated, therapeutic commodities could be, and indeed were, bought directly by the patients as well as dispensed by medical practitioners.[66]

The colonist's medicine chest, therefore, was symbolic of the expansion of the British therapeutics trade in the Empire. This web of transnational trade in industrially produced therapeutic commodities from the metropolis was facilitated by the iconic 'medicine chest' that could be customised for size, contain the latest tabloids or old and familiar pills and powders, replenished when depleted, and supplemented by local substitutes and alternatives, if necessary. In this sense, the various British firms' branded medicine chests represented enduring British imperial influence. More materially, the medicine chests represented industrial, branded therapeutic products that possessed remarkable portability, differentiating these commodities from the products of the older drugs trade. Enduring reputations were built on the basis of personal representations to medical practitioners with the aid of local dealers and salesmen. In 1933, for instance, medical representatives from B.W. & Co. wrote how a doctor in Sydney had only to check the brand on the label to immediately agree that the (new) product under discussion was bound to be effective. Medical practitioners from distant settler colonies wrote to the firm's headquarters in London to praise the quality of their products, sometimes decades after they were dispatched from London.[67] It was not only the medical chest that travelled to Africa and Asia from London but also the promise of scientific and modern medicine itself.

Yet the British and Anglo-Indian consumer was only one part of a much more diverse and complex medical market. Beyond the glittering British retailers' showrooms in Calcutta and Bombay, Simla and Kanpur, lurked the 'bazaar market' populated with Indian importers who dealt in British, German, and Swiss therapies; Japanese umbrellas and ointments; and Italian toiletries. They negotiated substantial discounts from the British importers for their goods, at the same time as underselling them with cheaper imports from the Continent. They distributed local therapies manufactured by Indigenous firms and participated in similar marketing strategies as the British importers by heavily advertising in the English and regional language presses, distributing flyers and circulars, and even canvassing medical practitioners. Inevitably, British importers viewed them as interlopers and often as fraudulent chancers at the same time as they also partnered with and traded with many of them. The British and the bazaar market were inextricably linked. The bazaar traders were joined at the turn of the century by increasing numbers of Indian producers of Western as well as Indigenous and non-Western therapies who provided further competition to the British-Indian distributors and manufacturers.

2

The Bazaar and the Indigenous Pharmaceuticals Industry

The colonial consumer was not a homogenous figure. The medical market in India reproduced the hierarchies and complexities of the subcontinent's social relationships. Medical consumers ranged from the British and the local elites who bought expensive, imported, patented, and branded medicines to desperate customers who bought powders and potions for a few pice from spice sellers and drug peddlers. This market was segmented but it was not mutually exclusive. Through the network of agents down to the local towns and remote outposts, and the mail-order system and the modern communication and transport links in the colonies, the international drug companies reached the homes of the emergent Indian middle classes. The medical market, moreover, was one of the most intensely contested sites of nationalist politics. The debates over the legitimacy of Indigenous versus Western medical systems ranged not just between the practitioners of the different medical systems or in nuances within official discourse. Medical consumers were divided over these too. In the late nineteenth century, most industrial manufacturers of drugs, whether Ayurvedic or Unani, or homeopathic or allopathic, claimed scientific authority and adherence to scientific processes in their medical commodities. The bazaar market accommodated all sorts of consumers and manufacturers of diverse backgrounds and differing capacities.

In this context, a handful of Indian manufacturers challenged the dominance of the British-Indian distributor/manufacturers within a nationalist framework by establishing laboratory-based, self-consciously Indigenous pharmaceutical manufacturing units that aimed for industrial self-sufficiency in colonial India. The historiography of Indian science and industry locates the Bengal Chemical and Pharmaceutical Works (est. 1893) in Calcutta, in particular, and the Alembic Chemical Works Limited (est. 1903) in Bombay as examples of the pioneering scientific pharmaceutical firms. Historians see these firms as representative of successful initiatives of science-based, nationalist industrialism. Their trajectories in colonial India are similarly understood as representing the paradigmatic structural limits faced by the Indigenous industry in colonial India.[1] A more nuanced interpretation locates the struggles and modest expansions of Indigenous chemical/pharmaceutical industries in the lack of technological innovation, capital, and international networks and government patronage that were available to British and American firms.[2]

Structural limitations and lack of government support hobbled the expansion of both firms in the inter-war years. However, rather than seeing them as isolated and pioneering scientific laboratories that promoted Indigenous industry, this discussion locates both firms within a larger network of Indian manufacturers/distributors who comprised the bazaar market in colonial India. This chapter will look at the Indigenous component of the medical market and argues that Indigenous firms that were laboratory-based and scientific in outlook were structurally similar to 'bazaar' firms and manufactured and marketed much of the same commodities. Therefore, the practical application of nationalist science in India did not engender radically new medical therapies. Instead, the Indian firms competed in the same market as the British, American, and German manufacturers as well as their British-Indian counterparts who were distributors and manufacturers. The Indian firms were disadvantaged in being identified as the 'bazaar' end of the market by their British counterparts and struggled to access government patronage or official legitimacy in colonial India.

The 'Bazaar Market'

Beneath the price range and luxurious displays in the Europeanized commercial streets of British India there lurked a large "bazaar" market, catered to by Indian distributors and wholesalers. In the first decade of the twentieth century, these had proliferated in number and occupied a large share of the market. Indeed, as an editorial in the British trade journal *The Chemist and Druggist* pointed out,

> The drug-trade is changing but slowly, that is to say, the strictly English pharmacies do not multiply, as they are needed solely by the white people and richer natives. The bulk of the people get their medicines from the bazaar druggists, who are becoming more numerous. They are keen buyers, because they are the keenest sellers in the world. Their buying is very largely done on the spot, a number of English firms having so comprehensive representation that the best that is going is quickly snapped up. German firms are now keen competitors, especially for certain chemicals, and do direct business with the bazaars.[3]

The large numbers of middle- and lower-class urban Indians were catered to by the 'native pharmacists'. This broad category of pharmacist was numerous; they encompassed the occupational descendant of the spice merchant who provided 'bazaar medicine' to the large-scale importers and distributors of European pharmaceutical products. The latter even competed directly with the European pharmacies, often with great profit for themselves. Occasionally, they negotiated with British importers to distribute their products and imports as well as Indigenous manufactured goods. The agent and proprietors of Burroughs Wellcome. and Co., for instance, were enraged when they discovered that British importers in Madras, the agency house of W.E. Smith and Sons, were passing on a part of their 'unique' discount for certain branded products to the Indian distributors, H.S. Abdul Gunny and Co., of Calcutta. Their agent sent stern warnings to stop the practice, but in a diverse marketplace, even the British distributing partnership companies moved beyond their European niches to participate in the 'bazaar' trade in pharmaceutical goods.[4]

While the European, largely British, pharmacies mostly imported pharmaceutical products from Great Britain, the Indian distributors were more flexible and resorted to importing from the rising industrializing nations of Germany, the USA, and Japan at cheaper rates for similar products and could, thereby, undersell British drugs. As a visiting American pharmacist noted in the late nineteenth century, this was a constant irritant to British distributors in India: 'The patent medicine trade is large, but it is much hampered by the natives, who sell at prices that Europeans cannot touch'.[5]

In 1892, the *Indian Medical Record* estimated that in Calcutta alone, there were around 756 druggists divided into three grades – those lit by electricity, those with beautifully presented showrooms, and the crowded wholesalers in the native bazaars.[6] Bombay had a similarly large number of Indian druggists-cum manufacturers. The Indian chemists, who generally depended on a larger volume of sales and lower profit margins, were flexible about their supplies and willing to import products from outside of Great Britain, especially if the prices were cheaper. Although they largely catered to different sections of the market, there was fierce competition for the non-proprietary section of the market between the large European pharmacists and local Indian druggists. The European pharmacists generally alleged that several 'bazaar' pharmacists bought adulterated and inferior medical products 'cheap bazaar catch-lines from Great Britain'.[7] Indian traders favoured German products because of the flexibility and the attention they afforded to the market. As an Indian resident in England pointed out, the British traders needed to 'adapt himself more to the requirements, tastes and prejudices of the millions in India', just like the German exporters.[8] These included attention to details in the market, from narrowing the size of marrow spoons to suit the size of Indian sheep to selling whole canned fruit, keeping in mind the Hindu taboo of not eating fruit cut by people of a different caste.

Not just the German manufacturers, American manufacturers too outdid the British in marketing to Indian bazaar traders. Although the British export of drugs and chemicals to India remained dominant, by the 1920s, these held only about half of the total value of imported drugs. In 1918, for instance, the director of agriculture and industries in Punjab pointed out how the non-British manufacturers from the Continent and North Americas expanded their markets in India:

> The establishment by large manufacturing Firms of Agencies and Sub-Agencies to exploit every little bazaar-this the Foreign firms have taken full advantage of while the British representative too often ignores them. These Agencies give facilities for viewing samples and accept the smallest order which is shipped along with larger consignments.
>
> … The shipping of goods on combined Bill of Lading offers a great inducement, not only does it save expense in shipping charges but it enables retail firms to renew stock frequently in small quantities without

> incurring extra charges of minimum freights, dock charges, insurance … These orders not only a mount to large sums in the aggregate but help to popularize and advertise the goods. The American is strong on this system. A bolder and more enterprising propaganda is necessary on the part of the British Trade representative which would reach the smaller dealers who cater for the masses … the Britisher considers his time too valuable to waste in the Indian bazaars.[9]

Although it is not possible to quantify the worth or value of the medical market in the 'Indian bazaars', the British-Indian distributors and traders were acutely aware of the competition. As well as from American and German firms, competition came from Indian bazaar traders and often overlapped with their trade. The Merchandise Marks Act (Act IV of 1889) in India was aimed at discouraging bazaar traders from importing commodities from Germany, given the prevalent assumption that British commodities ensured the best quality and were prized above others by consumers in the bazaar.[10] It was soon considered almost impossible to police merchandise labels in the ports. For instance, in 1889, when the Bombay-based firm of Kemp and Company imported eighty-five cases of port wine manufactured in Portugal routed through London, these were labelled as simply 'Fine Old Matured Invalids' Port, Kemp and Co., Bombay'.[11] The Government of India concluded that the firm's argument that the European origins of port wine were 'generally known' and the labelling not intended to deceive was correct, but also that it would be 'impossible to hit importers intending to deceive without touching others who had no such intention'.[12] And so it proved. Almost fifty years later, R.N. Chopra who chaired the Drugs Enquiry Committee (1930) pointed out publicly that the Act of 1889 could be used to penalize 'mislabeling' of trade names but was rarely used to control the adulteration of drugs, which was facilitated by manufacturing firms in Britain and the Continent that continued to produce medicines and therapies of inferior quality specifically for the 'bazaar market' in India.[13] The bazaar, therefore, although a heterogeneous marketplace, represented both the cheaper and the less salubrious end of the medical market and was more often than not associated with Indian traders.

In the last decade of the nineteenth century, the expanding market in therapeutic and cosmetic commodities also made possible a large non-British share of the Indian medical market, both from within India and internationally.

Many Indian drug sellers, particularly the wholesale druggists, began to manufacture their own products including patent and proprietary medicines, especially the ubiquitous fever, cholera, and dysentery pills. One of the largest firms in India, B.K. Paul of Calcutta was both an importer and producer of medicines. It began as a small family firm and by 1905, this company employed around three hundred assistants in their retail outlets in Calcutta alone. For a time before the First World War, B.K. Paul even enjoyed the 'the distinguished and (to a Bengali) rare honor of Viceregal patronage' of the governor of Bengal.[14] The family firm of B.K. Paul manufactured their own proprietary, patent, and homeopathic medicines and surgical instruments; they also imported and distributed pharmaceutical products from Europe and North America. Their main retail establishment in Calcutta rivaled in display any other European agency. Their bid to secure a royal warranty in 1919, however, failed, but after the expansion of the company during the First World War, they employed over fifteen hundred workers.[15] The grandson of the founder, H.N. Paul, formed the first short-lived professional body of pharmacists, the Calcutta Chemists and Druggists Association, immediately after the war, which lobbied for favorable exchange rates from British banks in Calcutta.[16] The firm of B.K. Paul was featured in the medical trades directories for wholesale druggists published in Britain, along with Wellcome Burroughs, Boots Pure Drugs Company, and Parke, Davis and Company and the British-Indian companies of Smith Stanistreet and Company and D.S. Kemp and Company of Calcutta and Bombay respectively.[17]

There were other large Indian drug sellers, especially in Bombay, for instance, where Indigenous capital had a freer rein than it did in eastern India. N. Powell and Company was established in c.1889 by an Indian, A.L. Nair. His company traded in imported pharmaceuticals and surgical instruments and manufactured surgical instruments. In 1909, he was the only non-European importer and distributor who exhibited his products at the exhibition of the Bombay Medical Union; by this time, his company was the Indian agent of several exporters as well.[18] N. Powell and Company led the informal association of Bombay chemists and druggists, especially speaking on behalf of the Indian merchants.[19] After the First World War, the proprietor toured Britain and the Continent to canvass for agencies from British exporters.[20] At this time, the Company provided medical instruments to the J.J. Hospital, Bombay.[21] In the 1930s, the company (along with better-known firms such as Alembic Chemical Works Limited and Bengal Chemical and Pharmaceutical Company) was commended as the producer of the best quality surgical instruments, asthma tablets, cod liver oil, chlorodyne, cough medicine, kidney pills, liver pills, lung tonic, health salt, quinine tablets, and sundry tinctures and tonics, all of which could, the Bombay Medical Union declared, replace imports.[22]

N. Powell & Company were respectable and presumably had a satisfyingly large clientele that enabled them to sustain their business. Their British trade name, meanwhile, provides a clue to the networks and bias intrinsic to the import and distribution of therapeutic commodities that may have lasted until the 1930s. It was not unusual for Indian traders and manufacturers to register their firms with an English name. This was a source of continual complaint from British merchants who alleged that such nomenclature was adopted by Indians to profit fraudulently from the justified reputation for fine quality enjoyed by British commodities and correspondingly the good credit on trust offered to British traders. This too was allegedly a bazaar practice.[23] In 1922, the Government of India sent out circulars to all provincial governments asking them to solicit their merchant associations' opinions on legislation compelling all partners in firms to disclose their 'own' names. This was in response to repeated complaints from the Anglo-Indian press and British-dominated merchants' associations in Calcutta, Madras, and Allahabad. It proved to be a complex issue. The Bombay Chamber of Commerce strongly supported and provided examples of this practice in Bombay and the Calcutta Trades Association asserted that 'the practice is of long standing, and it may latterly have considerably increased'.[24] But Indian traders robustly resisted any such legislation, pointing out that often British traders sold their entire firm including the name and the goodwill associated with it with the clear understanding that the 'goodwill', in this case, the racial advantage of an English name, would be used in perpetuity. The fact that the clarity over trade names and ownership was a conflict over keeping racial advantages secure is clear enough because officials and British trade associations agreed that only owners with 'Asiatic' names who traded in English-sounding trade names be subject to the relevant legislation, ignoring, for instances, the Portuguese who 'Europeanised' their names. Therefore, the bazaar market, although deeply entangled with the high-end British firms, often partnering with them and acting as their distributors in the mofussils, remained racially marked with

Indianness as well as with moral dubiety. When Indian nationalists began to manufacture and market Western medicine in the Indian cities, they attempted to brand their products as distinct from those of the stigmatised bazaar, although they were not entirely successful.

Swadeshi Nationalism and the Bengal Chemical and Pharmaceutical Works

Meanwhile, rising nationalist aspirations from the late nineteenth century highlighted the economic exploitation of the colonial state. Nationalists were concerned that the cost of industrialization in England was the decline of manufacturing in India. They advocated economic nationalism; with large-scale protests at the partition of Bengal in 1905, the Swadeshi movement invited the boycott of foreign goods as well as supported Indigenous manufacture. Although the Swadeshi industries established in Bengal between 1905 and 1911, generally by prosperous gentlemen zamindars, failed to sustain themselves, economic nationalism remained a great force in Indian politics and economy throughout the nationalist struggle. Several Indian chemical and pharmaceutical companies were established between 1900 and 1907. These were founded by, or employed, chemists who were trained in scientific techniques and interested in setting up laboratories that would manufacture pharmaceuticals of the B.P. standard to compete directly with imported pharmaceuticals.

The Bengal Chemical and Pharmaceutical Works (BCPW), celebrated in independent India for its pioneering pharmaceutical production, expanded in the inter-war years and competed directly with British and American firms as well as the British-Indian distributor and manufacturing pharmacists. Emergent Indian pharmaceutical companies competed for the same market and manufactured both 'Western' and Ayurvedic medicines. Firms like Alembic Chemical Works Ltd (ACWL) did not retail their products like the older agency houses and family firms but instead concentrated on the distribution of their goods wholesale to all of India. They also took the opportunity to display their products at industrial exhibitions in India, especially once the Swadeshi movement for economic nationalism gained momentum.[25] The manufacturers in the soaps, chemicals and perfumery, and confectionary sections all provided Indian alternatives to imported chocolate, tinned milk, and soaps, as well as patent medicines and numerous drugs with the added attraction of reduced prices for the middle-class urban consumers.[26]

Both the new industrial pharmaceutical companies like the BCPW and ACWL, as well as the older importer-manufacturers like B.K. Paul, won awards at Swadeshi industrial exhibitions for the best quality products in therapeutic goods.[27] The nationalist activism of P.C. Ray of BCPW and to a lesser extent, of Tribhuvandas Kalyandas Gajjar (ACWL) has served to highlight their importance in Indian industrialism in nationalist discourse. Historians have argued that they were both pioneers (and particularly Ray, a nationalist) of the pharmaceutical industry in British India.[28] It needs emphasizing here that Ray's and Gajjar's entrepreneurships were part of a broader trend that included the commercial world of manufacturers cum importers and dealers such as B.K. Paul and N. Powell and Company. There was a continuum, therefore, from the so-called bazaar dealers to the scientifically trained manufacturers that involved a host of importers, distributors, and producers. The new scientific and modern Indian drug factories were nonetheless distinct in one crucial sense; they clearly articulated nationalist aspirations and economic self-sufficiency in drugs.

The BCPW was established in 1893 by P.C. Ray, a Bengali chemist. Ray was educated at universities first in Calcutta and then at Edinburgh. He held a deep belief in the progressive power of industrialism. While teaching chemistry at the Presidency College in Calcutta on his return from Edinburgh, he aspired to use the natural products of Bengal to feed its impoverished population. He concluded that scientific industrialism was necessary through his reading of history: 'The history of the gigantic progress of industry achieved in Europe and America is a history of the triumphs of researchers in the laboratory'.[29] Simultaneously, after witnessing and working with famine relief organisations during recurrent famines in Bengal, he 'could not fail to notice what an immense boon the Charka could have proved to the starving people if it had not been abandoned nearly a century before'.[30] Following Gandhi, he advocated the *charkha* for the cause of economic regeneration in stagnating rural India.

BCPW started as a small-scale project with a modest capital of 700 rupees when Ray was still experimenting with his first products. His self-defined remit was to see how chemistry could facilitate industrial production. His

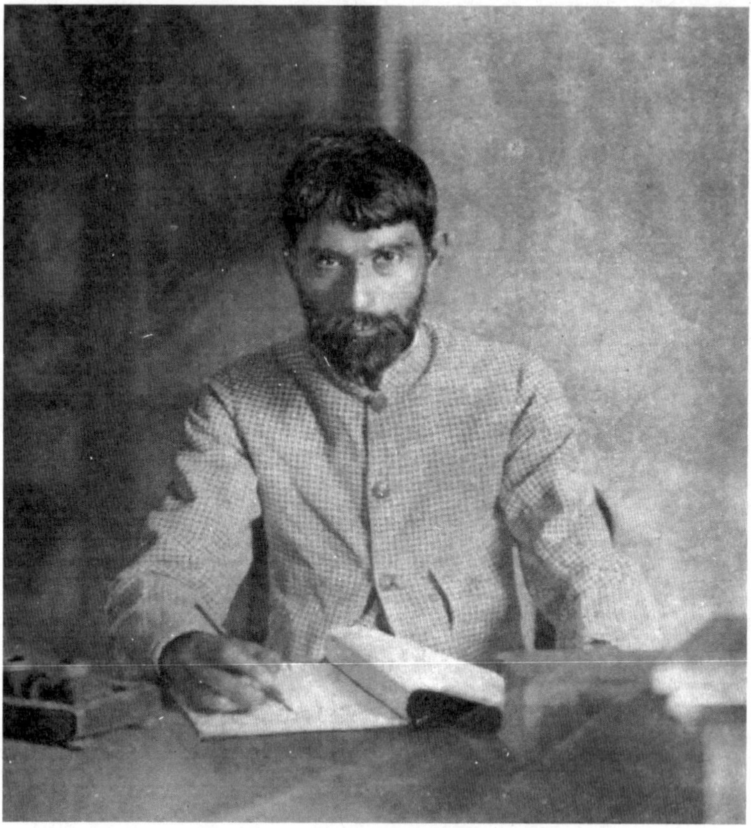

Figure 2.1 Photograph of P.C. Ray, 1909

first attempt at producing citric acid from lemon juice, although successful, had to be dropped as it was economically not viable.[31] Chemical industries required large capital outlay and infrastructure. He experimented with producing fine carbonate of soda (washing soda) from the local *saji mati*, but found that cheaper soda was available and the market in India and all of east Asia was monopolised by the British firm, Brunner Mond; similarly, he produced phosphate of soda from cattle bones scavenged from local slaughterhouses.[32] He soon realised that pharmaceutical preparations had a more ready market. He examined the numerous and varied Calcutta drugstores to find out about the quantities of drugs imported from Britain and found that most of the British pharmaceutical drugs that were available for sale in India comprised galenicals (medical preparations that are made from plants or animal tissues, rather than being created synthetically) and could be produced without much difficulty.

As we have seen in the previous chapter, the medical marketplace in colonial India was intensely competitive. As the first avowedly scientific pharmaceutical firm, self-consciously distinct from the British-Indian manufacturer/distributors or the drug/spice sellers of the bazaars, the BCPW was a metaphorical David against the Goliath of British capital. The BCPW began with the production and sale of simple galenicals. Even to manufacture these he had to first manufacture basic chemicals like sulphuric acid in his modest workshops. He consulted with Bhutnath Paul of the firm of B.K. Paul, who assured him that B.P. standard therapeutics would be assured of ready sales.

However, when Ray's sole salesman began to market bottled and labelled products to the drug sellers in the bazaar, they 'expressed their admiration but shook their heads saying *Bilati* (imported) drugs … command a ready sale, whereas *Deshi* (indigenous) drugs would be refused by our customers'.[33] Gradually, the quality of his commodities interested some bazaar retailers and found 'a back seat in the shelves of the local druggists'.[34] It was, however, through canvassing among prominent Bengali doctors in the hospitals of Calcutta who began to 'slowly and steadily' prescribe BCPW's commodities that brought the BCPW into prominence.[35]

Yet, the BCPW's productions were not limited to the BP. The firm manufactured Ayurvedic therapies, often in consultation with practising *kavirajs* in Calcutta. Ray recounts how his associates and friends, qualified Bengali doctors, first persuaded him to produce Ayurvedic therapies, prescribed them to their own patients, and encouraged Ray to experiment and improve upon old Ayurvedic formulae:

> I began with pharmaceutical preparations; but Amulyacharan gave a new direction to our business. He consulted several Kavirajas and collected from them formula and recipes for the Ayurvedic preparations, e.g., extract of Kalmegh (Andrographis pani-.-culata) ; extract of Kurchi (Holarrhena antidysenterica) ; syrup of Vasaka (Adhatoda Vasica) ; Aqua Ptychotis (Ajowan water) and placed them in my hands … he began a regular campaign in favour of these and impressed upon the profession the fact that the efficacy of these drugs had been proved beyond doubt

> by their universal use in the households of Bengal. Amulyacharan himself took the lead in boldly using these in his prescriptions. Slowly but surely they began to creep into favour and well they might. It was the universal practice in those days to prescribe syrup of tolu as an expectorant; but it was found that syrup of Vasaka acted more efficaciously. Our newly introduced Indigenous drug preparations thus began to make headway on their own merits.[36]

The BCPW's products were, therefore, cultural hybrids. Indeed, a reading of his autobiography affirms that Ray's seminar work, *A History of Hindu Chemistry,* was inspired by his interest in Ayurvedic formulae and Indian alchemical traditions originally gathered for the BCPW's manufacturers. The firm used local Bengali *bhadralok* contacts in the medical profession to popularise its products. Although the BCPW initially struggled to entrench its products to up-country retailers in the bazaar, the Bengali firm of B.K. Paul put in large orders for its products.

The import substitution needed by the Government of India during the Great War facilitated production by not only the BCPW but several other pharmaceutical companies that sprang up at this time. By the 1930s, BCPW employed 2000 workers and their net assets amounted to around fifty million rupees. As far as Ray was concerned, the BCPW was not just a vehicle of industrial production and commercial profit but also an institution of social regeneration. India needed not just industrialization but modernization, which could come through the social application of science. Along with this drive towards a science-industry link, the BCPW was also conceived within a strong rhetoric of self-reliance; at two levels, first for the Bengalis as a social group and second, for the nation in need of economic regeneration.

But this boom was followed by a sudden decline in the post-war period when the industry was again faced with an uncooperative colonial regime. This was also the time when foreign companies were keen to regain markets lost during the war. The war led to the growth of massive capacities for chemical industries in the West. Since most of the industrialised countries were suffering from overproduction, those like the US, France, Germany, and England had closed their markets with high import tariffs. This only kept colonial markets like that of India open for foreign exploitation. By the end of the Second World War, the BCPW's markets stagnated due to a number of other factors as well: lack of government tariff protection for Indian industries, stagnation in Indigenous research, and excise import duties imposed by the Bombay and Madras governments that discriminated against industrial products from Bengal.

Alembic Chemical Works and Indigenous Enterprise

A second Indigenous and laboratory-based pharmaceutical firm, the ACWL, was established in western India by a former chemistry professor. In 1902, T.K. Gajjar, who taught chemistry at Wilson College in the city, started a small laboratory and workshop with his former student in Parel, the Indigenous industrial district in Bombay. As a chemistry professor, Gajjar had a trajectory similar to Ray's in some respects; however, his social background was distinct. M. Mehta has identified two distinct and parallel scientific strands in pre-colonial India; the elite Brahmins who monopolised knowledge and whose ideas were speculative and theoretical and the craftsmen from the 'untouchable' castes whose work was imbued with empirical and technological, scientific knowledge.[37] Mehta argued that Gajjar, who was from the 'Suthar' or carpenter caste, fell into the latter category. His family belonged to the Vaishya-Suthar caste in south Gujarat, which was a community that had a slightly higher status than those of ordinary carpenters because they followed upper-caste ritualistic norms and in addition to their craft also traded in timber. Gajjar's father was a prosperous timber merchant based in Surat and Ahmedabad, and an architect and sculptor. Gajjar, one of several siblings, did very well at school in Surat and then at the Elphinstone College at the University of Bombay, where he graduated in chemistry and obtained his master's degree.

After having been awarded his postgraduate degree, Gajjar, who proudly claimed his caste status and skills, attempted to set up a school of technology for the boys of artisan castes in Surat through a wealthy philanthropist. Unfortunately, this could not be realized because of the unexpected death of his prospective benefactor. This is where the history of ACWL became closely aligned with that of the princely state of Baroda and its technical institute, the Kala Bhawan. Although occupying two-thirds of the territory of the Indian subcontinent, the hundreds of princely (native) states under titular sovereigns

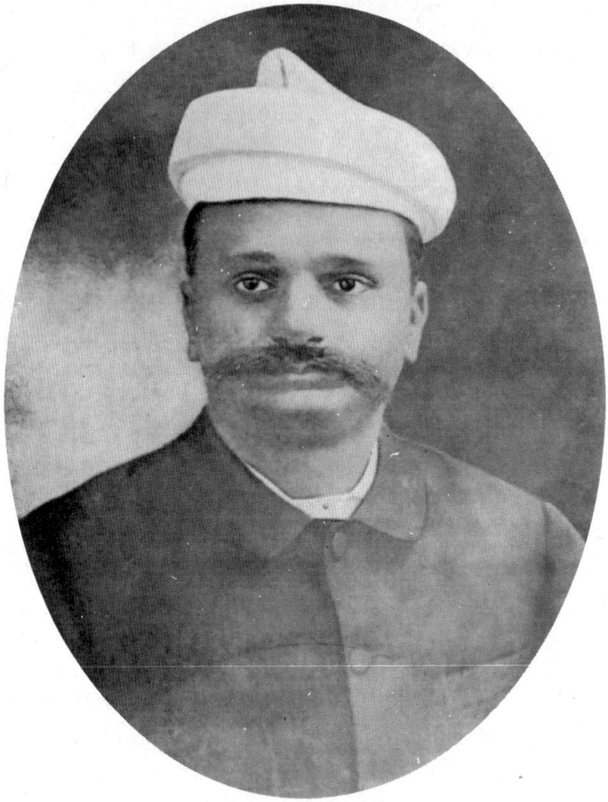

Figure 2.2 Image of T.K. Gajjar
(From A History of the Alembic Chemical Works Limited, 1939)

were controlled indirectly through British political agents and usually had little room for political or administrative autonomy. However, the state of Baroda in western India modernized its administration, streamlined its revenue collections, patronised Indian music and dance, and established the Baroda College based on the Western model of education under its celebrated modernist ruler Sayajirao III. The state started industrial concerns as 'models', providing the initial infrastructure, capital, and running costs.[38] Gajjar was invited by the ruler of Baroda, Sayajirao, to the professorship of chemistry in the newly set up university at Baroda. He soon persuaded Sayajirao to set up a polytechnic to harness the skills of young men of the craftsman castes in the state of Baroda. In 1890, the Baroda Polytechnic (Kala Bhavan) was established to train future industrial workers, with Gajjar at the helm of affairs. Within a few years, Kala Bhavan graduates were employed at industrial units in Ahmedabad and Bombay, but also in newly established industries in Karachi, Kanpur, Nagpur, Amritsar, and Calcutta. Alongside these Indigenous industrialization initiatives, in a long-term commitment to modern industrialism, the state established a department of commerce and industry, abolished import and export duties, and cleared policies to facilitate industrial concerns.

One of the industrial units was the state-owned Kala Bhawan workshops, which was given the contract to produce goods for the use of several state departments.[39] Within a decade, Baroda boasted of a total of 142 industrial units that included the production of cotton ginning, metal works, cotton presses, cutlery works, candle works and glycerine and soap, distilleries and chemical works, oil mills, sugar, ice, printing, slate, china clay, dyeing, chocolate, mortar mills, electric works, brush factory, and foundries, including the large production units at the Kala Bhawan workshop itself.[40]

By the time Gajjar quit the Kala Bhavan in 1899 in annoyance at the bureaucracy involved in running the establishment, around 800 students had been trained in carpentry, drawing, architecture, dyeing, and weaving, along with physics and chemistry. During this time, he avidly read current technological literature from Germany and translated these into Gujarati in a book titled *Rangarahasya* (Secrets of Colours). The Kala Bhawan did not live up to the promise of an Indian engineering centre that would facilitate and generate new and innovative technologies. Instead, its progress was in technical education, and it did succeed in providing a solid technical basis for the dyeing industry, and its students came to be chiefly employed in the textile mills of Ahmedabad and Bombay.

After he left Kala Bhavan, Gajjar went to Bombay and joined Wilson College as a professor of chemistry. It was in Bombay in that he established a Techno-Chemical Laboratory in Girgam, close to textile factories in Bombay where he used his skills to professionally clean pearls and offer consultancy on chemical dyes.[41] In the laboratory, he also trained students of chemistry. One of his students, A.S. Kotibhaskar, set up his own laboratory in Parel and began experimenting with making basic drugs and tinctures; he persuaded Gajjar to invest the substantial sum of Rs 50,000 in the venture. The firm was registered in 1899 as Alembic Chemical Works Limited (ACWL). Initially, the ACWL produced tinctures and galenicals, much like the BCPW. The firm expanded its

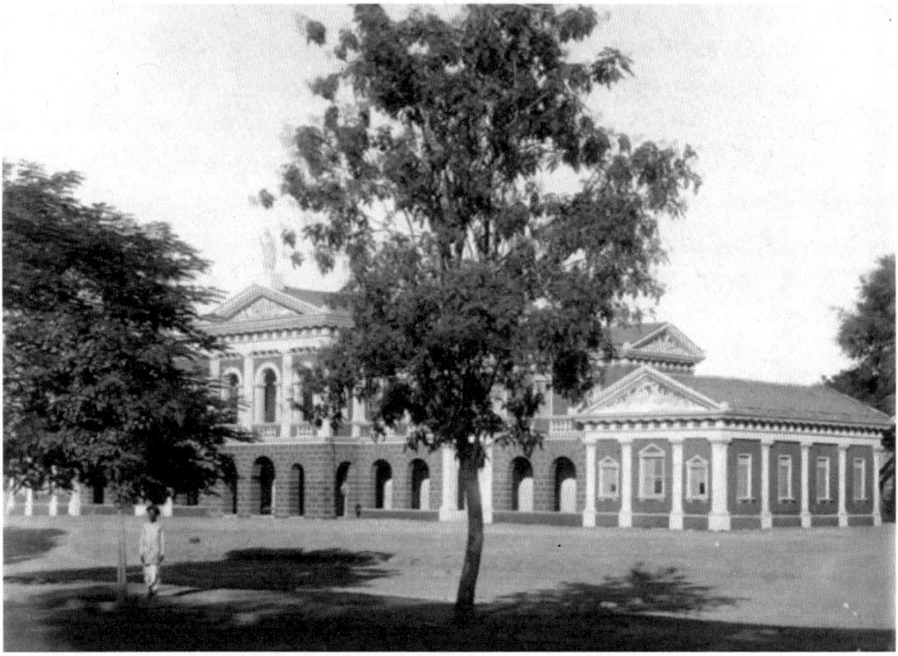

Figure 2.3 The Kala Bhavan, Baroda

range of commodities as well as increased its volumes of output and profit after it shifted from Bombay to the princely state of Baroda.[42] In 1907, Gajjar and Kotibhaskar were joined by Bhailal D. Amin. Amin was an entrepreneur whose family wealth was derived from agricultural land rather than from the traditional merchant communities. Amin and Gajjar decided to shift their company to Baroda and appeal to the philanthropy and modernist vision of Sayajiyao in establishing a pharmaceutical industry in his territories. Although the ACWL was registered in Bombay, it moved to Baroda in 1907. Here, the ACWL was granted free land outside the capital city for its factories. The Baroda government granted it a revenue holiday for ten years. The ACWL received added incentives for production, such as the construction of roads at the government's cost for the supply of goods from the factory to the nearest port, the supply of free water and sewerage facilities, etc. But the most lucrative aspect of the princely connection, so far as the firm was concerned, was that it received the exclusive contract to produce alcohol in the state of Baroda.

Nasir Tyabji has suggested some of the princely rulers enjoyed the trust of the British, which allowed them to pursue their economic goals independently, especially in comparison with the British-governed presidencies.[43] Although Tyabji has referred to native states within the Madras presidency, his point explains the limited industrialization and modernization of princely states more generally. Manu Bhagavan, on a different note, has compared the princely states of Baroda and Mysore to argue that princely industrialism was the product of a general thrust towards modernity, which included museums, Western education, and fragmented infrastructural developments.[44] David Hardiman had preempted some of these perspectives when he pointed out how the Baroda state under Sayajirao refashioned its agrarian revenue, finance policies, and, indeed, its collaborators to reinvent its sovereign as both enlightened and nationalistic.[45]

While streamlining its revenue, the Baroda government, following the British government, de-legitimized the production of fermented alcoholic drinks within its territories. The government in British India, by this measure, obliterated long traditions of home brewing in the country, principally because locally made wines and spirits were difficult to control, quantify, and tax, while the so-called IMFL (India-made foreign liquor – gin, rum, and beer) produced a large income through excise duties.[46] The Baroda government banned the local home-brewed mahua wine made from wild mahua flowers. Instead, it commissioned the ACWL to produce all the mahua–based distilled (not fermented) alcohol for sale in the entire princely state. This hugely increased the excise receipts of the Baroda government.

Although the ACWL began with manufacturing tinctures and galenicals and simple drugs for pharmaceutical use, its expansion came through the liquor contract from the Baroda state. The pharmaceutical business was soon eclipsed by the monopoly contract to produce enough liquor to supply the state-licensed distributors.[47] Moreover, the ACWL exported alcohol, particularly to the Bombay presidency neighbouring the Baroda territories and also to the metropolis of Bombay.[48] The princely connection helped ACWL in its excise negotiations with the provincial governments in Bombay, Madras, Calcutta, and Punjab. We have seen how Baroda's patronage of industries went from state-owned industries to state-subsidised industries. In the case of ACWL, the Baroda state also sanctioned the exclusive use of its pharmaceutical products in all the medical department's and hospital's purchases.

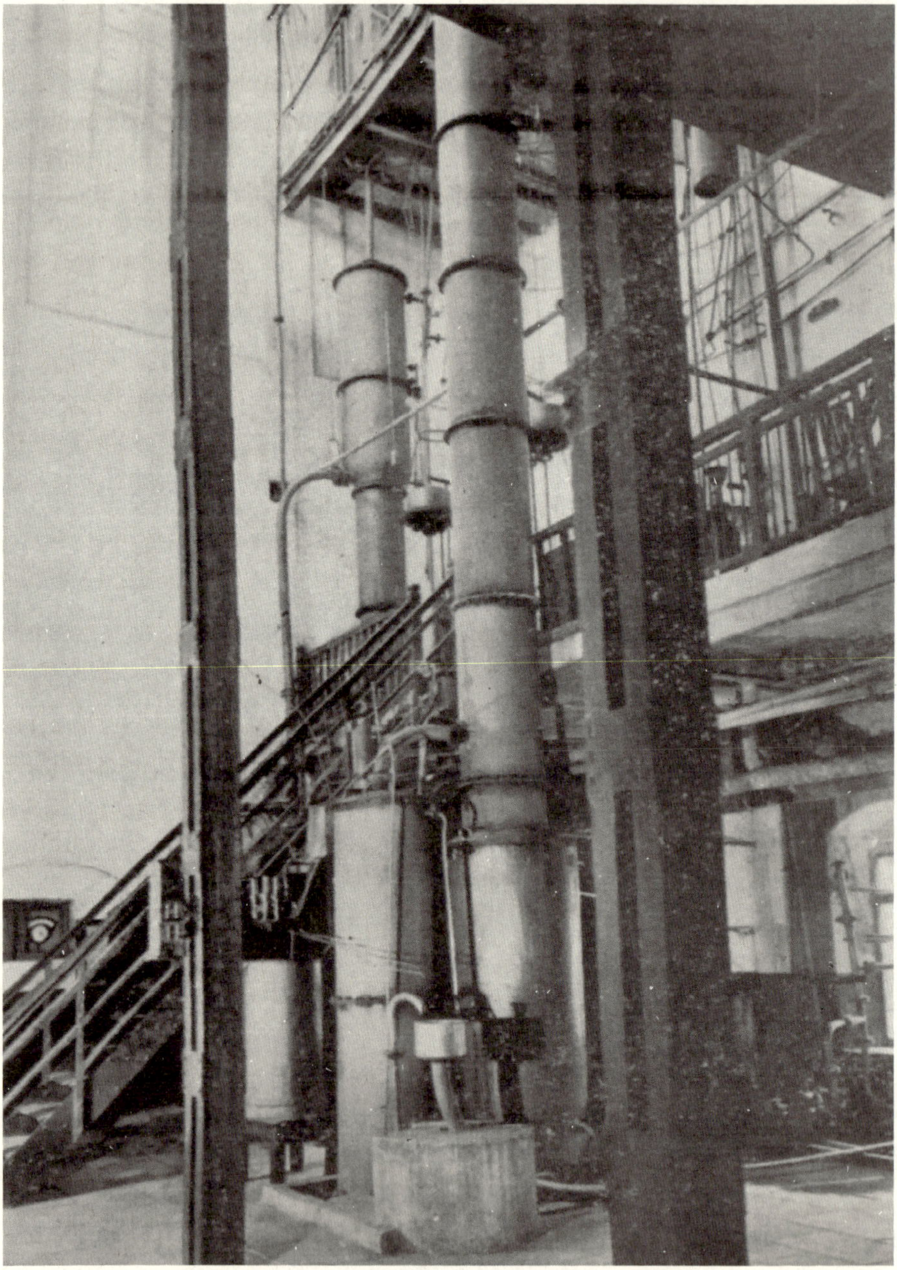

Figure 2.4 Ethyl Alcohol Distillery, ACWL, 2007

This prerogative of an assured market had formerly only been given to the state-owned Kala Bhawan workshops.[49]

With the First World War, imports of cheap German liquors, chemicals, and pharmaceuticals ended abruptly. This left the field clear to Indian suppliers, including the ACWL.[50] During the War, the fortunes of ACWL rose along with those of many Indian manufacturers of drugs, both Western and Indigenous. Several British-Indian and Indian manufacturing units of varying capacities produced and supplied surgical instruments, medicinal chemicals, acids, glassware, and industrial alcohol to the British army and the open market. As British trade and professional bodies pointed out in London, for instance:

> Now entirely manufactured locally ... loose woven bandages, absorbent cotton wool and yarn, etc., and gauze, double cyanide, compressed and uncompressed, carbolised and boric wool, and many forms of bandages, etc ...Whereas before the war, absolute alcohol-, refined petroleum, lysoaidyl, etc., and many of the preparations from belladonna, and nux vomica, were entirely imported, they are now being made satisfactorily in India. Thymol, ether for pharmaceutical purposes, quinine hydro-–chloridûm, acidum, strong ammonia, etc., are all now obtainable locally.[51]

After the War, however, the Indian market was inundated with British, American, and Continental therapeutic commodities of all kinds, patent and proprietary medicines, surgical instruments, and bulk generic drugs. The Indian pharmaceutical companies (including British-Indian ones) struggled to compete with them. However, while the BCPW, with P.C. Ray at its helm, struggled to compete with multinational companies within the context of unfair tariffs and intra-provincial excise duties, the ACWL could support its pharmaceutical branch through the reliable profits from alcohol manufacture and excise and tariff concessions from the Baroda state. B.D. Amin also used his closeness to the Baroda state to request tariff concessions from provincial governments in Punjab, Madras, and other regions within British India.[52] Between 1912 and 1938, the ACWL made multiple representations to the Government of India to ease tariff duties between provinces to facilitate its manufactures' transport across the entire subcontinent. It levied pressure through Indian trade bodies like the prominent and influential Indian Merchants' Chamber (headquartered in Bombay). The ACWL presented its case to the Indian Industrial (Holland) Committee of 1918, the Drugs Enquiry (Chopra) Committee of 1930, and the Tariffs Committee (1933). All of these were directed at what the firm viewed as unfair tariff rates imposed on exports of manufactured products from princely states into British India, including customs duties and excise on products containing alcohol. The firm also pointed out how railway freights as well as tariff rates benefitted importers of pharmaceutical preparations rather than Indian manufacturers. In fact, the Drugs Enquiry Committee (DEC) report (1931) recommended a reduction in the import duty of raw drugs into India used for manufacture by both British-Indian and Indian-owned firms, although the government did not respond to the suggestion. In 1938, the ACWL's letter to the Central Board of Revenue pointed out that, whereas, import duty on raw drugs and packaging material not available in India disadvantaged Indigenous manufacturers, inland drug manufacturers outside the presidency capitals of Calcutta or Bombay suffered greater disadvantages due to the railway freight charges on these articles. It showed that tariff anomalies enabled a raw drug from the local market in Orissa (seeds of nux vomica, used in the manufacture of strychnine) to be available at half the price in London than it cost to use in Baroda.[53]

Nonetheless, the ACWL was able to use its princely as well as nationalist merchant connections to gain monopolies and concessions that were beyond the means of other similarly placed manufacturing firms in other provinces and completely overwhelm new and smaller firms that manufactured similar products closer to its base in Baroda. The National Chemical Works Limited (NCWL), established in Navsari (located between Baroda and Bombay), was one Indigenous company that similarly manufactured galenicals and rectified spirits and competed with ACWL.[54] Its managing agent was one Gordhandhas Khushaldas Gandhi, and in 1934, its paid-up capital was a modest Rs 8,000. The firm claimed to manufacture hundreds of alcoholic tinctures (578 in total) in accordance with the formulae of the BP. Besides these, its catalogue of products listed toiletries such as hair oil, perfumes, shampoo, and around seventy-six proprietary medicines. Its products included a 'Malaria Mixture', a gonorrhoea mixture, the nerve tonic 'Nervatone', and a 'National Blood Purifier' prepared from several Ayurvedic drugs, besides standard Ayurvedic drugs such as *hartaki, kumara asava, maker dhvaj*.[55] In the 1930s, the NCWL made repeated requests to the Government of Bombay for tariff concessions similar to those ACWL had wrangled through the interventions of the Baroda Durbar. It also petitioned the Punjab, Berar, and Central Provinces for similar concessions without success. Lacking the advantages of tax concessions and monopoly contracts that ACWL could rely on, the National Chemicals Works Limited faded away.

Similar to the ACWL was the Mysore Government Soap Factory based in the princely state of Mysore, which like Baroda followed an industrial policy from the late nineteenth century onwards. The model of industrialisation here differed a little from Baroda in that the state owned the factories that processed the valuable local sandalwood. It began as an industrial unit to process sandalwood oil obtained from the extensive forests of the Mysore state.[56] During the First World War, export to Britain stopped almost entirely; less than 5 per cent of the 1313 tons of sandalwood offered for sale was exported in 1914–15. In 1916, the Mysore state established a sandalwood distillery in Bangalore.[57] By 1921, the products of the distillery, now called Mysore Government Soap Factory, included sandalwood oil and manufactured sandalwood soap. It also produced other high-value essential oils from local botanical material including cardamoms, rosha grass, lemon grass, and ajwain seeds, all of which were marketed under its own brand name.[58] By 1921, the princely state owned a host of industrial units, including a lamp factory, porcelain, steel works, etc. and supported several privately owned manufacturing firms through the grant of free land, loans, and state purchase of their products.[59] One such firm, the Bangalore-based Mysore Pharmaceuticals Limited, manufactured proprietary medicines, essential oils, and galenicals and was expanding its markets in British India. Their list of therapeutic commodities was a familiar mix of drugs and formulae borrowed from Western and Indigenous systems, including a 'Cholera Diarrhoea and Dysentery Compound' besides 'Distilled Waters Decoctions Eau de Cologne Elixirs Emplastrums Essences Extracts Essential Oils Glycerines Infusions Liniments Liquors Lysol Medicine Chests … Polishes Powders Spirits Syrups Tablets Tinctures Unguents'.[60] It obtained the usual government subsidies and protection within Mysore. The firm was able to market its therapeutic commodities in provinces in British India by having the Mysore government settle its logistic problems with railway freight rates, and even had the Mysore government act as guarantor for the accurately noted alcohol content in their tinctures for tariff purposes in British India.[61]

In 1935, it registered as a limited company with a paid-up capital of one lakh rupees. The firm was aided by the Mysore state's commitments to establish institutions for curative medicine, including hospitals, sanitary Western-style medical education, and training in Ayurveda and Unani.[62]

Indigenous Drugs Manufacture and 'English' Medicines

Two intersecting trajectories shaped the histories of firms such as the BCPW, ACWL, and others. On the one hand, they were examples of the new breed of scientist-nationalists emerging through the university system and their laboratories who committed themselves equally to the nationalist cause and scientific production of B.P.-grade therapeutic products. On the other hand, these firms were closely linked to the manufacture and selling of Indigenous drugs emerging from the Indian bazaars.

While both BCPW and ACWL flourished initially, the competition with imported drugs and chemicals was unequal. In the absence of regular state patronage, BCPW eventually floundered; its fortunes rose briefly in the Second World War, but its research into new drugs and extension into distant markets stalled. Meanwhile, ACWL also found it difficult to compete with foreign competition, but as its alcohol-producing unit received regular patronage from Baroda state, as did its entry into the alcohol and the drugs market in the entire Indian subcontinent, it was able to sustain both ends of its production. Once the Second World War began, ACWL was prepared for the rush in the expansion of production of drugs through increased capacity and its own manufactory for making glass bottles, which other manufacturers had to import. ACWL used its opportunities and emerged, at the end of the war, as a premier Indigenous research-based pharmaceutical manufacturing company. In independent India, it claimed to be the only manufacturing firm to eschew foreign collaboration and could boast of having designed and established its own antibiotics manufacturing plant.[63] The protection offered to established Indian industrialists in Nehruvian India that, according to Tirthankar Roy, skewed Indian industrialisation, enabled ACWL to diversify its manufactures and extend its markets.[64] ACWL's deft use of lobbying through nationalist and trade organisations such as the Indian Merchants' Chamber and its ability to access government support from the princely state and then from successive postcolonial governments helped it to attain its present iconic status as an established, even iconic, pharmaceutical firm.

Apart from the provincial and national lobbying, sustenance for firms such as BCPW and others came from the tradition of Indigenous drug manufacture connected to the bazaars of India. This was in the hybrid nature of the drugs they manufactured and marketed. A spectrum of various manufacturers, from BCPW to Zandu Pharmaceuticals Limited (henceforth ZPL) to B.K. Paul, made their presence felt in both sectors of the disparate drugs market in India. Scholars of Indigenous medicine have demonstrated how Ayurvedic and Unani medicine manufacturers packaged their medicines and successfully advertised proprietary medicines widely in the new print media in the late nineteenth century. Their repertoire of proprietary medicines and specifics also expanded.[65] From the mid-nineteenth century, Indigenous therapies for cholera increased in numbers, as did the recurrent epidemics.[66] Unlike malaria or plague, British medical men had little knowledge of the dreaded disease and were often willing to try Indigenous therapies for cholera. The expansion of Indigenous drugs and their availability in volume and variety was owed to the expansion of the medical market itself from the late nineteenth century. Although it is not possible to quantify these, there is no evidence that the demand for therapeutic commodities shrank during the lean periods of depression in the 1920s or at any time later. Drugs and therapies in every form were in demand in urban India and Indigenous medicines and their practitioners participated in the boom. Many proprietary medicines were produced by individual vaids or hakims or doctors who actively practised medicine. Their packaged therapies usually carried their names often with their qualifications (real or fictional) and profile pictures prominently displayed. The most successful could use their reputation as exceptional medical men to establish workshops. These often continued as family businesses. For instance, ZPL, which was established in 1910 in Bombay by Jugatram Vaidya, began as a small firm manufacturing traditional Ayurvedic remedies. Jugatram was a grandson of Zandu Bhatt, a renowned and celebrated Vaidya who practised Ayurvedic medicine in the princely state of Jamnagar and had been the physician to the ruler. This family firm soon shared proprietorship with another family, the Parikhs, to enable them to expand the business and invited several others into the partnership in 1919.[67] The firm was very successful by the 1930s when it established additional factories near Bombay. Like all such family firms, ZPL used regional community-based networks to market its commodities. Distributors from the Gujarati and Bania communities were offered tempting bulk discounts and other benefits in regional urban centres. In the 1930s, they directly sold their products in retail like most other manufacturers. The firm had a large retail store in Kalbadevi where the Indian commercial area or 'bazaar' was located in Bombay.[68] Twenty-six agents in Bombay city and its suburbs (all Gujarati Bania family firms) stocked its products, which they sold in drugs and pharmacy stores, general grocery stores, and specialised spice sellers.[69] ZPL also commissioned thirty wholesale and retail agents in the Gujarat and Kutch regions, including family firms, individual vaids, and even one doctor.[70] The ZPL claimed that traditional vaids and hakims as well as 'western medicine practising doctors' used their therapeutic products.[71] Like other pharmaceutical firms in urban India, it advertised heavily in the regional press and published its own books on home remedies and materia medica. It declared that most of its customers were 'middle class' and that the firm was committed to reducing the burden of the cost of medicines for everyday use for its consumers.[72] Predictably enough, although the firm emphasised its distinctiveness as Indigenous and even Swadeshi medicine manufacturers, (the fiery and popular nationalist Tilak visited their Bombay factory) they also produced and advertised 'English Medicines' including 'Zandu Malt Extract B.P.', cod liver oil, and 'syrup of hypo-phosphate'. The firm produced several cosmetic products, including scented coconut hair oil, 'parfum de Zandu', and 'Zandu Snow'.[73] Its reputation in manufacturing Ayurvedic medicines 'on the most up to date' methods was referred to in the Drugs Enquiry Committee report.[74] After independence it continued to expand its sales and range of products, which were stocked widely, especially in the cities and towns in western India. When ZPL was finally taken over by a competitor in 2008, of the original two families, the Vaidya family owned 27 per cent and the Parikhs 33 per cent of the shares of the firm.[75] Similar Indigenous medicine manufacturers that successfully marketed their products widely included Dabur, established in Calcutta in the 1880s by the medical practitioner S.K. Burman. Its best-selling commodities were hair oil and tonics, although it has expanded its range of products to patented medicines for several chronic diseases in contemporary India. Another equally well-known and popular firm and Unani medicine brand was the Hamdard Dawa Khana, established by Hakim Ajmal Khan, a prominent nationalist and institution builder. As historians have pointed out, Hamdard emerged from the recognisable family-based elite Unani practice in old Delhi.[76] Ajmal Khan, Congressman and vocal advocate of the modernization of Indigenous medical systems, transformed it into a formal medical college for both Ayurvedic and Unani medicine as well as a manufacturing firm. At the time of independence, Hamdard was the most popular manufacturer of Unani therapies in undivided India and its proprietary medicines continued to remain the most recognisable.[77]

Conclusion: The Pharmacy and the Bazaar

Recent scholarship has pointed out how Ayurveda and Unani reformulated themselves structurally through organized corporate bodies and restructured pedagogy in colonial India. These debates were intensely political, but they related essentially to the systems of medicine in a broader sense. The practice of medicine and the treatments delivered to medical consumers were much more eclectic. Historians have written of the persistence of subaltern medical practitioners in Ayurveda/Hakimi traditions whose knowledge and methods differed from the text-centric high cultures of medicine. Similarly, it has been shown how the practises in Western medicine have been vernacularised in colonial India; allopathy and homeopathy were received and adapted in the late nineteenth and twentieth centuries. Even within Western medicine, marginalized trends like mesmerism or hypnotherapy and its practitioners obtained some legitimacy and support, however briefly.

Scholars have also pointed out the corporatisation and the nationalist politics involved in the commodification of Indigenous medicines. What is to be stressed here is that these medicines were marketed as such, but were hybrid, heterogeneous, and cosmopolitan. The best-known medicine manufacturers self-identified as scientific, laboratory-based firms but these, such as the BCPW, ACWL, or ZPL manufactured and marketed a medley of therapies derived from Indigenous medicine and drugs as well as tinctures and unguents based on B.P. standard formulae. Their significance is that these were available for the consumer. Historians have referred to the heterogeneous Indian market, but their writings have emphasised the cultural and institutional changes in medical praxis and pedagogy in colonial India. Scholars have also pointed out how Indigenous medicine firms expanded their outputs and globalised selected commodities successfully in the contemporary context.[78] But as we have seen in this chapter, some manufacturers had scientific training, and others depended on a traditional, family-based reputation of knowledge and expertise. Nonetheless, the BCPW, ZPL, ACWL, and B.K. Paul and Hamdard, all manufactured similar therapies and proprietary medicines based on drugs and formulae from the B.P. and Ayurvedic and Hakimi texts.

The 'bazaar market', therefore, was a complex, layered one inhabited by a wide range of traders and manufacturers, from the small spice and drugs sellers to large traders who skilfully negotiated supplies from Germany, USA, and Japan, undercutting the more conventional and established British traders and distributors. By the early twentieth century, there were also significant Indian manufacturers of Western therapeutic and surgical commodities. With the emergence of an Indian industrial base for pharmaceuticals, the demands for an Indian pharmacopeia to replace the BP gathered momentum from the nationalist press as well as Indian medical men. This demand grew louder during the Great War when imports from abroad stopped almost entirely and there was a great shortage of medicines.

3

For a Pharmacopeia for India

The first Indian Pharmacopeia was published in 1955 after the establishment of the postcolonial nation-state.[1] This was the culmination of a long-standing attempt to create an Indian pharmacopeia by both Indian and British medical practitioners in British India. The demand for an official Indian pharmacopeia reflected the need for an official standard for dispensing therapies so that the potency and character of each drug used in specific formulations remained fixed and uniform. It did not represent the need for a compendium or a dispensatory of Indian drugs, of which there were several.[2] This chapter captures the quest for this elusive standard in the disparate Indian medical market.

Unlike in Western Europe and the USA, where pharmacists were professionalized in the nineteenth century and standardized their respective pharmacopeias, there was no such process evident in colonial India. This is not to say that the pharmacopeia of Great Britain, Germany, or the USA did not change or evolve after their formalization in the mid-nineteenth century. Newer editions continued to be published that included new drugs and innovative formularies and were incorporated into the standardized pharmacopeia of the respective nations.[3] In colonial India, meanwhile, the formalization of a standardized pharmacopeia was a fractious and complex affair that did not achieve fruition until after the Indian Independence.

As we have seen in the previous chapters, 'bazaar medicines' were used extensively by European surgeons and physicians in the Indian subcontinent since the seventeenth century. The use of these continued well into the twentieth century, and in any case, as the previous chapters have shown, the term 'bazaar medicine' itself was so broad and eclectic that it encompassed a vast range of therapies not only of Indian origin but those drawing from older, Eurasian trading and knowledge networks.[4] At the same time, it was the BP that held sway as a legitimate, albeit informal, pharmacopeia of colonial India. In the absence of any drug legislation, the BP served as the unofficial but unquestioned standard for all therapeutic commodities in British India. Since the BP standard was unofficial, its use in formulae by manufacturers or pharmacists was discretionary and could not be legally enforced until the Drug Acts of 1940. This enabled drugs and therapeutic preparations of disparate standards and quality to be sold legally by a heterogeneous range of pharmacists and medical practitioners.

The wide disjuncture between the legitimate standard for therapeutic commodities and the products on sale in the market was a source of disquiet to Western-educated Indian doctors, and even, to an extent, to the predominantly British personnel of the Indian Medical Service (IMS). After all, most practitioners of Western medicine regularly used well-known Indian drugs and formularies. Later, once the Swadeshi movement (the nationalist movement to adopt Indian products as opposed to Western ones) gained traction ideologically in nationalist politics in the early twentieth century, the question of the substitution of cheaper, fresher, and more readily available Indian drugs for expensive imported ones assumed commercial significance as well as political urgency. Therefore, the campaign for an Indian pharmacopeia was not just a nationalist issue. It was advocated for by state administrators intensely convinced of the need for parsimony by the government in British India and supported by a section of officialdom within the IMS as well.

After the *Bengal Dispensatory* was compiled in 1844, Edward John Waring's *Pharmacopeia of India*, commissioned by the Secretary of State for India in the aftermath of the 1865 BP, served to acquaint medical officials in India with the common bazaar drugs available in Indian markets and functioned as a semi-official compilation.[5] This did not, however, fulfil the need for an official standard in the Indian medical market. This was yet another compendium of drugs, as was Waring's *Bazaar Medicine*, published a few years previously.[6] A more significant intervention was the attempt by the Pharmaceutical Association in Britain to include a list of Indian drugs in a supplementary addition to the BP of 1898.

This supplement, compiled as a concession to the use of Indian and other non-European medical materials by the military medical establishment in India and a campaign by a vocal section of Western-educated Indian medical men, was titled the 'Indian and Colonial Addendum' to its main BP of 1898 and published separately in 1901.[7] It included fifty-five formulae from Indian medicines. The 'Indian and Colonial Addendum' led to a fierce debate on the need for an Indian pharmacopeia in medical, official, and public discourse in colonial India. There were two points of contention. The first was the inclusion of Indigenous drugs, both Unani and Ayurvedic. Opponents of the Indian pharmacopeia argued that most of the drugs in the addendum were of historical or exotic value and that Indigenous drugs were too numerous and their quality and potency too uncertain and untested to merit their inclusion in an official pharmacopeia. Those in favour of an Indian pharmacopeia countered that the British medical establishment used Indian drugs widely but denied the necessity for an official Indian pharmacopeia to facilitate the import of British and American drugs within the large and lucrative Indian market.

The second was the identity of Indigenous medicine itself. Several drugs originating in India were traded, prescribed, and used in India and globally. These included the ubiquitous opium in various forms, as well as the widely used nux vomica, essential oils of cinnamon and clove, and by the twentieth century, *chiretta* and *chaulmoogra*, which were processed and marketed in India by transnational firms such as Burroughs Wellcome and Bayer. Were these to be regarded as 'Indian' drugs or, once legitimated by the BP, did these transcend the boundaries (and the taint) of being Indigenous medicine? These prompted the emotive question: What validated Indian drugs? Furthermore, what legitimised Indigenous systems of medicine?

The debate around the Indian Pharmacopeia became an ideological conflict that blended science with cultural and economic nationalism. No pharmacopeia of India was formally compiled and legally made mandatory until after independence. This chapter investigates the impossibility of an Indian pharmacopeia in British India. This impossibility was located at the site of the validity of the hundreds of Indian drugs in the market. These had to be identified precisely, cutting through the confusing nomenclature in different regional languages. The potency of each drug had to be tested and its active components isolated. In the crowded, eclectic, and uncertain bazaars in India, this proved to be a gargantuan, and ultimately, impossible endeavour. This chapter locates this impossible quest within the cultural, economic, and scientific debates around legitimacy, standardization, and economic imperialism.

Bazaar Drugs and the Indian Materia Medica

A wide array of Indian drugs used by traditional Indigenous practitioners were listed, categorised, and published from the time of the first European colonisations of India. This knowledge of Indian drugs included information gathered from Ayurvedic practitioners and hakims who were trained from the classical Ayurvedic or Unani texts as well as from the more numerous herbalists and spice sellers in the bazaars. Garcia D'Orta's *Simples and Colloquies of India* was the first of these.[8] Richard Grove has highlighted that D'Orta's compilation served to link botany and pharmacology more closely and introduced a host of drugs (around eighty) to the European world.[9] Indeed, as Patrick Wallis has pointed out, in Britain, for instance, the number of apothecary shops increased exponentially and the extent of their wares widened immeasurably in the seventeenth century.[10] Many were from the New World, but the easier and regular access to the Indian Ocean trading networks enriched the apothecaries' resources too. When Hendrik Van Rheede, the Dutch governor in Kerala, published the twelve-volume *Hortus Malabaricus* at the end of the seventeenth century, it represented, at multiple levels, the economic power of the Dutch empire as much as it did the entrenchment of empirical botany in the Western scientific world. Grove has argued that the botanical gardens and the 'experiments' that occurred in transplanting south and southeast Asian botanical materials and knowledge across the globe to European, principally Dutch metropolises, represented a cognitive marginalisation of the older Sanskrit and Arabic textual knowledge. In this process, he concludes, these transplantations were infused with a 'deeply Indigenous' character by collecting and privileging botanical information from local and low-caste collectors in southern and southwestern India.[11]

The use of Indian or 'bazaar' drugs by Western medical practitioners was eclectic, the East India Company surgeons often making do with the Indigenous drugs used by practitioners of all Indigenous traditions that were available for sale in the local markets. From the seventeenth century onwards, the

East India Company surgeons regularly used bazaar drugs in their practice, and these were supplied to the army and later, to civil hospitals as they were institutionalised in the colonial port towns of Madras, Bombay, and Calcutta.[12] The reasons were pragmatic; local drugs used in the hospitals were substitutes for drugs from Europe that had been either lost or destroyed, or their contents and potencies degraded in the long transit from Europe.[13] This practice resonated with the historical European experience of trading in the Indian Ocean where the intra-Asian trade had enriched European coffers as much as long-distance maritime trade had between Europe, Asia, and Africa.

While apothecaries and subsequently the pharmacists regulated their profession and standardised a pharmacopeia in the Western world, in India, the codified formularies of Indigenous drugs were initially an Orientalist enterprise that both scrutinised Indigenous 'classical' texts of Sanskritic origin and simultaneously codified and reified ancient texts.[14] B.S. Cohn and Lata Mani who (along with several others) studied Orientalist scholarship in nineteenth century India pointed out how the grand projects of the translation and codification of Indian systems of knowledge, governance, and morality privileged the elite, literate, and upper-caste communities and the Brahmins and Qazis who were the custodians of knowledge in pre-colonial India.[15] The Orientalist relocation of Indian epistemologies marginalised local knowledge and everyday customs and traditions that represented the lived experience of a vast proportion of Indian communities.

A parallel trajectory was a more diverse project consisting of the compilation of Indigenous drugs that were circulated in the regional and local drug markets, usually by East India Company botanists/surgeons interested in the potential of import substitution. Whitelaw Ainslie's *Materia Medica of Hindoostan*, published in 1813, for instance, introduced hundreds of local drugs available in the Madras presidency and used regularly by Indian and Western medical practitioners.[16] This was the first of several volumes of the materia *medica*, both regional and nation-wide, compiled and published in British India in the nineteenth century.

Historians who have worked on Indigenous drugs in colonial India have generally focussed on the 'reinvention' or the 'revival' of the institutions of Indigenous medicine, whether Ayurvedic or Unani.[17] Panikkar, Hardiman, Berger, and Sivaramakrishnan have shown how, when confronted with the challenge of Western medicine and its institutionalisation by the colonial state,

Indigenous practitioners organised themselves into corporate bodies.[18] The vaids and hakims used the rich and varied print cultures of regional languages and English to participate in the public sphere in the nineteenth century.[19] They politicised their epistemologies and posited them in conflict and competition with Western medicine.[20] In the process, they placed Ayurveda and Unani at the centre of nationalist debate on the validity of Indian epistemology and more broadly, the survival of Indigenous culture faced with an existentialist threat from the disjuncture occasioned by colonialism. The recent scholarship on Indigenous medicine, rich as it is with historical insights, has explored the histories of Ayurveda and Unani in colonial India in terms of their institutionalisation and corporatisation. Scholars have traced the trajectories of the associations of Indigenous medical practitioners, empathised with their conflictual relationship with the colonial state, and institutionalised Western medicine and their ambivalent intimacy with Indian nationalism. They have highlighted how Indigenous medicine was both homogenised and dynamic in responding to the encroachments of Western medicine on the livelihoods and social status of vaids and hakims, who were often dismissed as 'quacks' by the British and Indian Western medical practitioners.

However, there has been little scholarly attention to the drug market and its structures. Did the medical market in colonial India negotiate 'indigeneity' as a cultural *and* a commercial category? What were the implications of the demand for an Indian pharmacopeia in the market? Why did this demand for an Indian pharmacopeia persist throughout the late nineteenth and twentieth centuries in colonial India, and what were the political and economic consequences of this sustained demand?[21] I would argue that the need for an Indian pharmacopeia must be situated within nationalist politics and in the medical market in colonial India. The demand for an Indian pharmacopeia was driven by the need to understand and eventually standardise the Indigenous drug market, which would in turn legitimise the Indigenous drugs industry. The impossibility of the Indian Pharmacopeia is linked to the unfeasibility of that undertaking.

I have argued in chapters 2 and 5 that until the twentieth century there was little difference between the drugs used in Western medicine and Ayurveda and Unani, except in the processing and packaging. The new and articulate conglomerates of vaids and hakims in late Victorian India addressed themselves to these. They bottled their drugs and produced them in pill form industrially. They were attentive to branding and resorted to creating patent medicines. They borrowed from various Western medical traditions, drugs (e.g., cinchona), and techniques (e.g., counting the pulse, delivering injections); invested in advertising; and participated in the public sphere on the politically volatile subjects of Indigenous health, diets, and diseases of the newly emerged 'modernity' of urban Indians.[22] They fused their disease frameworks with heterodox Western systems (e.g., naturopathy, hydropathy).[23] In brief, they modernised their profession and interpreted the colonial subjectivity of the modern Indian self. The dualities of Western and Indigenous medicine, meanwhile, were sustained in the politics and commerce of colonial India.

The Many Pharmacopeias of India

In this context, it is evident that there were different and distinct demands for an Indian pharmacopoeia in medical, as well as in public discourse, in India. Even after the Orientalist paradigm was eclipsed, the publication of a plethora of compilations of Indigenous drugs continued in the nineteenth and twentieth centuries. Whitelaw Ainslie's work, with its textual and epistemological certitude, can also be read as the beginning of the textual marginalisation of Indigenous drugs. In addition, this marginalisation occurred at the level of the dispensers of these drugs. Projit Mukharji has argued that 'subaltern herb gatherers' were marginalised by Indian drug traders and pharmacists at this time.[24] Similarly, Rachel Berger has argued that Indian drugs in general were written out of the pharmacopoeia by the late nineteenth century.[25] This approach does not explain the retention of the various bazaar medicines in formularies such as John Waring's *Remarks on the Uses of Some of the Bazaar Medicines and Common Medical Plants of India* published in 1860. Waring's *Bazaar Medicines* proved enormously popular and made four editions by 1883. The first edition had been bilingual, in Tamil and English, printed for issuing to local vaccinators in the Madras medical establishment. Local vaccinators also functioned unofficially as both medical practitioners and medical informants on local medical materials until the late nineteenth century. The third edition, published in 1875, expected these formularies to be used widely in India and even in the Malay Straits. Thus, it is necessary to read Waring's 'bazaar' as the site of the praxis of Indigenous drugs; praxis, therefore, is key to explaining the emergence of the Indian Pharmacopeia.[26]

Perhaps this trajectory of an Indian pharmacopeia will be clearer with an analysis of Kanny Lall Dey's more modestly conceived compilation. Dey was a Western-educated physician and a much respected member of the first Indian Medical Congress. His *Indigenous Drugs of India: Short Descriptive Notices of the principal medicinal products met with in British India* was first published in 1867, then revised and re written in 1896. This represented his life long aspiration to collect, categorise, and finally, to fully integrate as many Indian drugs with Western materia medica as possible. Dey was the only Indian nominated to the first of many committees by the Government of India to make a comprehensive list of Indian medicinal plants in the first all-India Indigenous drugs research committee established by the Government of India.[27] In 1899, the *Chemist and Druggist* dismissed the endeavour to integrate Indigenous medicines within the British Pharmacopeia:

> So far, the committee has been little else than called into existence; it has met and corresponded, but does not feel clear as to what it is all about, or how it can benefit mankind by investigating things that are well known, so practically no useful end appears to have been served by the committee.[28]

This is apparent from a study of William Dymock's compilation. After Ainslie's work, the next voluminous addition in English to the Indian materia medica was William Dymock's *Pharmacographica Indica.*[29] This was a four volume magnum opus, and a follow up of his *The Vegetable Materia Medica of Western India,* published a decade previously. Dymock's volumes were a huge, collaborative attempt to document the botany of the Indian subcontinent as comprehensively as possible. Dymock was exceptional by the late nineteenth century. J.F. Royle, whose *Essay on the Antiquities of Hindoo Medicine* privileged ancient Indian medicine as historically preceding Greek and Arabic medicine (in an evolutionary paradigm), nonetheless, confined his collection of 'Hindoo' materia medica to materials within the London Pharmacopeia (1851) and the

British Pharmacopeia (1864).[30] There was a practical reason: the Bengal Board had commissioned Royle to compile a list of drugs available in the Indian bazaars that might be conveniently used as substitutes for the more expensive imported items. Royle's *Essay on the Antiquities* listed around 1000 botanical and mineral items sold in Indian bazaars as country medicines.[31] In his *Manual of Materia Medica and Therapeutics*, which went through several editions through the nineteenth century, Royle made it clear that his previous work was relevant to the extent that the histories of some drugs 'investigated by Hindoos' and used in the present could be identified.[32]

The volumes of Dymock's *Pharmacographica Indica*, unlike that of Royle's compilation, reveal more interesting ways in which the materia medica of India was evolving systematically towards a framework of pharmacological knowledge that would eventually be divested from its social and cultural roots. Therefore, historiographically, Dymock poses a problem. Can we take Dymock's account of 'mythological' and 'historical' Indian drugs as proof of Western engagement with Indian drugs, particularly in the context of their globalisation? Dymock's *Pharmacographia* claimed that the collection had put together scattered publications on the Indian pharmacopeia, often from obscure sources and had 'endeavoured to collect and verify this information, and supplement it where deficient by original investigation especially … the chemical composition and physiological action of the plants and drugs'. So far, Dymock seems to have been in line with the general trajectory of dissociating drugs from their broader contexts into chemistry oriented formularies. British physicians and pharmacists, including surgeons appointed at the government medical hospitals, still used 'bazaar' or 'country' medicines when European drugs were not available at the time of the publication of the *Pharmacographia*. There is no doubt that Dymock's *Pharmacographia* was used regularly by pharmacists and drug merchants in nineteenth- and early twentieth-century India. *The Chemist and Druggist* referred to Dymock's work to emphasise replacing belladonna with the indigenous *datura fastuosa*, a relatively new substitution. This, I suggest, was a different kind of substitution from the eighteenth-century bazaar substitutes used when European drugs were not available – it involved a deeper ingraining of the Indian drugs market with the global demands, and this was accepted by British authors of pharmacopeia. This deeper integration of Indigenous drugs indicated a new globalisation of Indian drugs.

As Kanny Lall Dey suggested in 1884, Calcutta had the potential of being established as a 'drug emporium which would be central to the great markets of the world'.[33]

Yet, there is a disjuncture here. The preface to the *Pharmacographia Indica* itemises unexpected materials that are difficult to fit into the above-mentioned trajectory. For example, 'Plants of historical and mythological origins' write the authors, 'are not omitted, as the history of Indian medicaments would be incomplete without them'.[34] This presents us with a difficulty: Was Dymock's collection a pharmacopeia or a history of materia medica in the Indian subcontinent? Why did Dymock include 'plants of historical and mythological origins'? He confirmed that these 'though possessing little or no medicinal activity, have not been omitted, as the history of Indian medicaments would be incomplete without them'. At the same time, Dymock articulated his wish to engage contemporary (Western) medical practitioners with his collection and provided comparisons of 'empirical estimates' of drugs with modern pharmacological research. These included a lengthy list of poisons as well as obscure drugs that were not used by Indians, such as the *Meconopsis Wallichii,* which did not have a vernacular Indian name, or the *Kaff Maryam*, imported from Syria and whose efficacy the author appears to have had no opinion of.[35] One possibility is that by enumerating the 'mythological' or 'historical' drugs, Dymock sought to both demystify them as well as emphasise their mythological nature. As for 'historical' drugs, cataloguing them comprehensively served to highlight their contemporary irrelevance beyond their value as Orientalist curiosities. In that regard, Dymock's work emerges as a historical record or an emporium of Oriental drugs more than a contemporary formulary.

These various pharmacopeias of India that were published by British scholars in India, such as those by Royle, Waring, Dymock, or Birdwood's extensive 'Economic Products' series, were compiled and published to meet the functional needs of an administration that was consolidating itself in the vast Indian subcontinent.[36] Nonetheless, these pharmacopeias proved to be of uncertain utilitarian value. They introduced Indian drugs to the English-speaking world and global trade. They offered information on substitutes for imported drugs and identified areas where raw botanical drugs were available naturally or could be cultivated systematically on a large scale. With the information collected from a dense network of informers within the subordinate medical service and a slew of collectors, drug sellers, and a motley group of medical practitioners from the bazaars, most of the formularies highlighted the multifarious drugs found regularly in the Indian markets. This compilation of knowledge of Indigenous drugs for use by Western medical practitioners was facilitated by scholarly engagement and by the need to explore potential resources in the colony that could be exported and processed in the metropolis in a classical colonial relationship. However, their value was supposed to be in the information they provided on the potential for substitutions for European drugs with Indigenous ones that could be used regularly and extensively. Therefore, while the burgeoning collections of materia medica of the Indian subcontinent were comprehensive and listed between 300 and 500 drugs, it was the drugs' potential for import substitution that would determine if they would be used regularly. The compilations of Indian materia medica proved to be less practical guides to making up prescriptions than grand statements of intent.

Towards the Definitive Pharmacopeia

The publication of several materia medica and formularies of Indian drugs highlighted the usefulness of Indian drugs for practitioners of Western medicine. Pharmacopeias were used as textbooks in the pharmacological curriculum of the medical colleges instituted by the government in Bombay, Calcutta, and Madras. As Indian medical graduates proliferated in private practice in urban centres, the so-called bazaar medicines often served them and their patients. Although British military/civil medical practitioners remained reluctant to use Indian drugs, the Indian medical community had fewer reservations. As K.D. Basu, an Indian doctor who had served in the subordinate medical service pointed out:

> The use of the Pharmacopoeia [of 1868] as a text-book in the colleges and schools of this country, has also been productive of some good … The native remedies having been rendered familiar during the period of studentship, have been often made use of by the full- fledged Indian Medical graduates.[37]

When the first Indian Medical Congress (IMC), an association of Western medical practitioners, was formed in 1894, it had a separate panel on pharmacology. Kanny Lall Dey, who was also the chemical examiner to the Government of Bengal and President of this section in IMC, strongly urged the government to explore the possibilities for the greater use of Indigenous drugs within the government/military hospitals in India and save the great expense of importing drugs from Britain or America. He recommended 'medical farms', 'drug emporiums', and laboratories to facilitate the cultivation and global marketing of Indian drugs. His promptings reflected a growing realisation among medical men, especially the now substantial section of Indians trained in Western medicine, that Indian drugs had the potential to become cheap, easily accessed, and even familiar alternatives to many staples that were imported at great cost from abroad:

> The gradual progress of Indian pharmacology, the widening and deepening of its influence, and its possibilities in contributing to the health and consequent prosperity of this vast Empire have been in complete sympathy with the gradual development of commerce, medicine, and science in this country … Clear of the mythology and superstition from which, not unlike the medical science of Europe it evolved, but which lingers still in India, the science has in some measure at least demonstrated the marvellously liberal pro-vision of curative and remedial agents within the reach of the teeming millions of this Empire.[38]

Subsequently, in 1896, the colonial government, always keen to tightening budgets, instituted an official enquiry into the Indigenous drugs of India, with Dey as an honorary member of the committee.[39] Among the three principal members of the committee was the Scottish botanist George Watt who had compiled the six-volume *Dictionary of the Economic Products of India* published between 1889 and 1893. The Committee submitted annual reports for three successive years and cited a few possible substitutes for European drugs while listing common drugs available in the bazaars but recommended little else that was significant. The *Chemist and Druggist* suggested that the project was based on the whim of a single individual, and pursued aimlessly:

> It was proposed in a moment of enthusiasm by Rai Bahadur Kanny Lall Dey … who, however, is too old to do the work himself; and others do not quite know what Dr Dey wants.[40]

The commercial interest of transnational pharmaceutical companies in sustaining the discourse of the non-availability or the uselessness of native remedies is obvious. British firms were favoured by the Government Medical Store, which was also the single biggest buyer of imported medical supplies and supplied the military and many civil government hospitals with medicines. At the turn of the century, British pharmaceutical companies faced stiff competition from German and USA firms whose products were cheaper and whose medical representatives were more innovative and enterprising than the agents of the traditionally dominant British ones. The exponential expansion of the private drug market and the decision by the government of India to not supply most civil medical institutions with free medicines from 1890 represented an opportunity for the relatively lesser-known and enterprising distributors of Continental, American, and even Japanese therapeutic commodities. It is understandable, therefore, that British firms or their trade journals would disdain any attempt to categorise and use Indigenous drugs in government hospitals and dispensaries in India.

When the Colonial and Indian Addendum to the B.P. of 1898 was published in 1900, although it contained fifty-five drugs of Indian origin, its reception in Britain was lukewarm. The *Lancet* anticipated that the addendum might 'do their part towards welding together the colonies and dependencies by supplying information relating to the modifications of treatment which are frequently necessitated by local conditions'.[41] Meanwhile the official British in India were even more dismissive. The *Indian Medical Gazette* was scathing about the substitutions offered in the Addendum:

> Such suggestions … of 'alternative substances' are … a dangerous innovation … Sesame oil and Aracliis oil are very good bland oils, and if in India they may be employed, well, as substitutes for olive oil, where is the line to be drawn ? Question if many of the drugs will meet with any general recognition even in India and the Colonies.[42]

The *Indian Medical Record*, which usually voiced the opinions of the subordinate medical officials who were Indians and accommodated the private practitioners of Western medicine, was more generous and optimistic about the addendum:

> Every experienced practitioner will frankly admit that the scientific recognition of certain Indian remedial agents … and their inclusion into the 'Imperial' Pharmacopeia, exhibits not only sound sense on the part of the British Committee, but it also places within the reach of practitioners in Great Britain and the Colonies a class of drugs that deserve a high place in the armamentarium of every unprejudiced healer.[43]

The private or 'independent' medical practitioners and lower-ranked medical officials in the government dispensaries who mostly treated Indians or the poorer British and Eurasians were not averse to trying out cheaper, local substitutes and using the Addendum as a practical guide. The *Indian Medical Record* even rued the absence of Hindustani names for the Latin ones in the list of Indigenous drugs that might have made 'the collection of such indigenous products easy for pharmaceutical collectors' and 'would have rendered this section of the BP far more interesting and useful to thousands of Indian practitioners'.[44]

The economic argument for an Indian pharmacopeia was straightforward. The colonial government, always parsimonious, favoured reliable alternatives that could be obtained closer and cheaper. Military medical men in charge of army and civil hospitals preferred, instead, imported British medicines at the cost of the government (and effectively the Indian taxpayer). Almost all the IMS at this time were educated in Britain; they sustained contact with 'home' and attributed sterling quality to all products manufactured in Britain. They went 'home' on furlough every few years, at which time they renewed their acquaintance with the agents of pharmaceutical companies. The colonial state allowed them private practice in their own time, but their patients comprised either the non-official British community or elite Indians who would not cavil at the cost of imported medicine and would fetishize commodities produced in European metropolises.

Therefore, despite a tenacious discourse of tropicality that persisted in colonial medicine well into the mid-twentieth century, privileging the view that tropical bodies were somehow different (from European/non-tropical bodies) and would respond better to drugs cultivated in the tropics, most drugs used in the government hospitals and dispensaries were imported.[45] The case for an Indian pharmacopeia was made by a handful of British officials, although they were vocal and articulate in public discourse. It was the Indians who trained in Western medicine, served in subordinate medical services, and were appointed to civil or military positions that consistently raised the demand for an Indian pharmacopeia. Their opinion, picked up and echoed as well by the Indian press, remained similar throughout the nineteenth and twentieth centuries. In this respect, colonial officials and Indian nationalists appeared to agree, although the requisitions by the Government did not expand to include Indian medical products except during the two world wars.

The second part of the economic argument for an Indian pharmacopeia that emerged was that it would enable the systematic cultivation of drugs in India and not only generate self-sufficiency but also provide substantial revenues from the commercial cultivation of Indian drugs. Although the systematic cultivation of drugs in India was not undertaken on a large scale (except cinchona and opium) by the government, there was little dispute that it was a thoroughly commendable aspiration. The only parties that were offended by all of this were the transnational firms, their distributors and sales agents in India, and the section of British medical men who continued to believe only in imported therapeutic products.

Impurity and the Problem of Standardization

The epistemological and political arguments for the publication and dissemination of an official Indian pharmacopeia, however, was another matter. Many British medical officials who were in charge of the hospital administration of the colonial state believed, with varying degrees of conviction, that Indigenous drugs were useful and that skilled vaids and hakims could and did perform a great service to the Indian public, particularly in the rural areas.[46] Their objections were to the 'impurities' within the drugs and the obfuscations, material and metaphorical, that were pervasive within the formulating, dispensing, and trading of Indigenous drugs.[47] The very plenitude of Indigenous drugs available in the bazaars, their immense regional variety and nomenclature, and the enormous difference in the status and scale of their dispensers and sellers occasioned deep disquiet among British medical and official administrators. This complex mistrust was projected through the tropes of purity/adulteration and efficacy/inefficacy.[48] The bulk of Indian drugs, they believed, needed to be collected and chemically examined, and their active principles investigated and demonstrated, before they could be usefully compiled in a pharmacopeia. The great variation in the quality of the drugs and their efficacy were impediments to the formal publication of an Indian pharmacopeia.

Even when they were engaged in identifying Indigenous drugs that could be usefully and cheaply introduced to Western medical practice, the variety of the products appeared to subvert their efficacy. As early as 1876, under an episodic tightening of budgets that the India Office in London enjoined on its administration in India, the Committee on the Supply of Drugs in India supported the publication of an Indian pharmacopeia, 'while the BP should remain the authoritative guide to all Medical Officers in India so far as drugs not Indian are concerned, an Indian pharmacopeia – truly such – should be prepared, treating only of drugs peculiar to India'.[49]

However, the Committee, comprising medical experts in Britain who were advised by Joseph Hooker himself, also contemplated that despite or perhaps because of the plenitude of drugs in the bazaars, the resultant pharmacopeia:

> might be of very modest dimensions … for it should include only drugs of proved utility, and should give the information regarding them in a very condensed form, including name, method of preparation, doses, therapeutic uses, comparable European drugs … The Committee desire to record a strong opinion against the introduction into this Pharmacopeia of many of the numerous useless drugs which enter so largely into the Materia Medica of Native practitioners of the old style: they contemplate a small practical work which shall plainly set forth those Indigenous drugs of knowledge and established value which are fitted to replace European drugs now sent out.[50]

Therefore, the formulation of an Indian pharmacopeia was intimately linked to the question of the efficacy of the various Indigenous drugs, although not always of the legitimacy of Indigenous systems of medicine. In the new century when both Indian nationalism and the consumption of imported drugs in Indian cities were conspicuous, the director general of the Indian Medical Service, Pardey Lukis, pointed out that a scientific approach to Indigenous drugs would enable their inclusion into the Western system of medicine, which itself had only recently accepted the germ theory of disease:

> I may say also that I do not recognise any fixed line of demarcation between the Eastern and the Western systems of medicine. The main difference … whereas one has advanced the other has remained stationary, and that is why I am an advocate for the placing of the ancient and indigenous systems of medicine upon a scientific basis … we are ourselves only just emerging from the slough of empiricism … I was almost howled down when I tried to deliver an address on the germ theory of disease before a Students' Debating Society.[51]

The pillar of 'scientific basis' on which Indigenous systems/drugs were to be reinstated within the established, government-aided medical institutions had proved elusive. The very first Central Indigenous Drugs Committee (established by the Government of India in 1896) had expressed clear reservations about the proposed Colonial and Indian Addendum to the Indian pharmacopeia and its members were sceptical about the vaids and hakims who had acted as the local informers for the project. The committee itself had declined the task:

> The members of the Central Indigenous Drugs Committee of India are unanimously of opinion that they are not at present in a position to formulate definite Statements as to the value of any indigenous drug, still less of a selection of such drugs. Further they do not believe that any previous Indian Committee, however constituted, could have been more able than they are, to make a selection of Indian drugs that could be authoritatively advanced as useful substitutes for the drugs of European Pharmacy.[52]

A stumbling block to the professed good intentions of utilising Indigenous drugs as cheaper and more easily accessible alternatives to imported products was that the drugs in the bazaar were not deemed reliable. This was both due to a lack of knowledge of the chemical components and active agents in many of these drugs and the perceived wilful fraud on the part of Indian drug sellers in the bazaars. When the English newspaper *Statesman* (Calcutta) began a campaign for a food and drugs law in India in 1911 to ensure the quality of drugs in the Indian market, it pointed out that 'many … medicinal preparations occurring in the Indian Bazaars are physiologically inactive, or others again are almost entirely deficient in active principle and are practically inert'.[53]

As we have seen in chapter 2, by the turn of the century, nationalist Indian scientists and industrialists had formed pharmaceutical companies in Indian cities. Indigenous medical practitioners, collectively through associations supported by nationalists, became bold and assertive on the legitimacy of their prescriptions. At this point, the identification of active principles became central to this legitimation. The Bengal Chemical and Pharmaceutical Works (BCPW), the pharmaceutical company set up by the Indian chemist P.C. Ray in 1897, manufactured therapies from Indian drugs and was one of the most successful Indian firms. The BCPW's trade booklet pointed out that although Indian drugs were included in the BP, they were not prescribed or popularised by the medical community 'because good and reliable preparations could not be procured'. The BCPW identified this as a great difficulty and declared:

> We have undertaken at this juncture the manufacture of medicines from Indian indigenous drugs … The preparations described in this book are prepared from selected mature drugs with the greatest care and skill to retain their full therapeutic value and have been placed in the market through trial. The drugs are collected fresh and in proper season and the manufacture is conducted under the supervision of trained and experienced chemists. Every preparation is tested in our Analytical Laboratory before it is sent out to the market.[54]

Vivian Quirke and Jean-Paul Gaudilliere have pointed out that the isolation of active principles of drugs revolutionised the drugs industry after the Second World War.[55] In colonial contexts, Pratik Chakrabarti and Anna Winterbottom argued that the identification of active principles resulted in analytical contractions where these were hauled out of their socio-cultural contexts and, further, an impoverishment of the materia medica because drugs of similar but not identical chemical content, used as alternatives, were marginalised and eventually disappeared from the markets.[56]

And indeed, identifying the precise chemical character of each Indigenous drug became central to the formulation of an Indian pharmacopeia. Unlike the compilations of materia medica in the nineteenth century, which listed hundreds of Indian drugs and their apparent innumerable variations, the Indian pharmacopeia needed to pass the test of scientific authenticity for each drug. This would not have affected the Indian drug market as the manufacturers in Britain, not to mention their competitors in Germany, the USA, and Japan, were ready and prepared to flood the newly emergent Indian market with their products. However, with the Great War and the stoppage of all imports from Europe and the USA, 'import substitution' and the formulation of an Indian pharmacopeia assumed immediate urgency. During and immediately after the Great War, British and Indian medical experts alike, in tune with the Indian public sphere in this, demanded an Indian pharmacopeia.

Meanwhile, the Indigenous medical practitioners, who had emerged as powerful conglomerates and politically affiliated with the nationalist movement, demanded formal recognition of their diplomas and the employment of the graduates from their new, Western-style colleges into government service. They also demanded the legitimation of their epistemologies and the patronage of their drugs from government hospitals. These conflicts, too, were mediated by the tropes of purity and scientific identification.

The Impossibility of an Indian Pharmacopeia

The promise of an Indian pharmacopeia in colonial India was at its brightest during and immediately after the Great War when the imports from the UK, Europe, and North America dwindled and then stopped almost entirely. Indian drug manufacturers expanded their operations and posted enormous profits, supplying the private market as well as government hospitals and dispensaries. However, this also accentuated the demand for cheaper and more accessible medicines, and, in the time of intense nationalist politics, resonated even in the nominated and circumscribed legislative assemblies. After several vocal demands in provincial assemblies, the Madras government commissioned a report on the efficacy of Indigenous drugs in the province to be conducted by M.V. Koman, a physician at the General Hospital in Madras.[57] Koman's report, written after consultation with hakims and vaids, was entirely dismissive of almost all the Indigenous drugs that he came across. The superintendent of Madras General Hospital told him that patients were refusing to be treated with the Indigenous drugs he had requisitioned and admissions to the hospital were falling due to his trials. Koman found nothing to convince him that either the texts or the practitioners could offer any useful knowledge or treatment not known to Western medical practitioners: 'In vain have I attempted to find any drug or medicine whose reputed marvellous properties are shrouded in mystery or are not already known'.[58] Although it caused an enormous furore in Madras and in India more generally, Koman's report served to squash pleas for government support to Indigenous medical institutions and, equally, to disparage attempts to establish Indian drugs within Western medical practice through an Indian pharmacopeia.[59] The *Indian and Eastern Druggist,* a trade journal published from London, gleefully pointed out that while 'it has been constantly urged in Indian medical journals and in pamphlets and other publications that the forests of India are rich in botanicals of medical value',... And that 'unwarranted claims have been made on behalf of the indigenous materia medica, and of the systems of medicine'.[60]

The colonial government, under intense pressure from the medical community and the public, instituted the Drugs Enquiry Committee (DEC) in 1929 to investigate the cultivation, production, import, marketing, and sale of the drug market in India. It was chaired by R.N. Chopra, professor of Pharmacology at the newly established Calcutta School of Tropical Medicine (1921). Chopra had begun his experiments into the efficacy of specific Indigenous drugs in the mid-1920s, the first sustained attempt to compile a 'scientific' Indian pharmacopeia. After the DEC report was published in 1931, he published his substantive *Indigenous Drugs of India* in 1933. At the Calcutta School, Chopra and his associates attempted to isolate the active principle/s of specific Indigenous drugs that they obtained from local markets. In doing so, Chopra and his associates (and indeed, every medical expert who referred to Indigenous drugs in India) subscribed to the Orientalist mythology of the 'ancient origins' and subsequent 'degeneration' of Indian (mostly Hindu) knowledge of medicine: 'History shows that many of our pharmacopeial drugs were known ... used in some form long before their use was introduced into the Western medicine'.[61] His approach was rigorously scientific; he sought to identify the active principle of the drug in question; if he could identify the active ingredient and prove its efficacy, he located not only the sites where it grew naturally but also areas it could be cultivated on a large scale. Therefore, the voluminous *Indigenous Drugs of India* was a powerful argument for the compilation of an Indian pharmacopeia on the grounds of the significance of *local* conditions of diseases as well as their cures:

> The altitude, the season, the climatic conditions … A plant showing remarkable activity in one part of the world may be inactive when collected from another … Again, there are racial variations in dosage … Each country should evolve a pharmacopeia best suited to its own peculiar climate and racial factors.[62]

The DEC report recommended regulating the market through a drugs act and stringent quality control on the production and advertising of Indigenous drugs (as well as laboratories to enforce standardisation of biomedical therapeutic commodities). A significant recommendation was the formulisation of an Indian pharmacopeia so that the vast potential of Indigenous drugs could be utilised to serve a stark demand for economical, safe, and effective drugs within India.[63] The DEC pointed out that India had historically maintained:

> such a fine old materia medica of her own that quite a number of the drugs used … should receive attention. A goodly number of these are identical in botanical origin with Western drugs, but the preparation of the crude material may not in all cases correspond with the standards laid down elsewhere. Other drugs may be chosen in order to give preference to a native species or a local product which, will be more convenient to obtain and more readily understood by the country at large.[64]

The Government of India implemented some of the recommendations of the DEC, including introducing a Drugs Bill, as late as 1940, when the scarcity of supplies from Germany and the UK made import substitutions a high priority. Through the 1930s, R.N. Chopra and his associates at the Calcutta School continued to painstakingly identify the botanical character of the bewildering varieties of Indigenous drugs one at a time and specify the particular efficacy and dosage of each. Although Chopra's *Indigenous Drugs of India* succeeded in identifying and making formulaic prescription possible for scores of well-known and a few relatively obscure drugs, the task of replicating this process with each Indigenous drug available in the bazaars was gargantuan, even impossible. As the *Madras Medical Journal* pointed out, even a relatively well-used drug like digitalis could pose difficulties:

> A large number of preparations of digitalis are on the market, purporting to possess all the advantages of digitalis without its drawbacks. Thus it is claimed for some of them, that, being pure principles, the dose is more uniform and the treatment more 'scientific' than when cruder preparations are employed. But … the active principles of digitalis are so little known that no two chemists working on them are agreed as to how many of them are present in the plant, and it may be question whether any one of them has been isolated. Much less are the preparations available for therapeutic purposes to be regarded as pure substances or an incorporating the whole virtues of digitalis. This would be of less moment if these so-called digitalines, digitoxins, gitalins and digalens were reliable in strength; unfortunately it has not yet been proved possible even for the same manufacturer working by the same method to put a uniform product on the market.[65]

While the seemingly Sisyphean task of scientifically demonstrating the efficacy of each Indian drug continued in the laboratories, an official, definitive Indian pharmacopeia could not be formulated or published. The nationalists railed against the government's iniquities and lack of attention to the needs of Indians who could not access essential drugs. The dreams of an Indian pharmacopeia never quite died down. The Indian pharmacopeia, along with the admittance of a greater number of Indians to the IMS and the institutionalization of tropical medicine research within India, rather than in the UK, were considered by Indian physicians to be essential for India's scientific and medical future. As the *Journal of South Indian Medicine*, a nationalist periodical for Indian medical men, pointed out in 1936:

> The compilation of an Indian Pharmacopeia is a great desideratum, and the time has now arrived for taking up this question in right earnest. The various formulae given in the British, USA and other Pharmaco-

> poeias may, after sufficient laboratory test and trial *in our own country*, be adopted with advantage and included in the Indian Pharmacopeia. The indigenous system of medicine may also be standardized and such of the therapeutic agents as are really efficacious may be brought within its fold. Let me repeat here, "If in the wake of the great enterprise of the study of Tropical Medicine, the examination of the IMS are held only in India, for the study of which candidates come here from the West, and if the Pharmacopeia of India be more Indian than at present, will that be an era in the history of medical science in India?"[66]

The vaids and hakims, regardless of general government indifference, validated themselves in the public sphere and were patronised by around two-thirds of the population, including sections of the affluent and well-informed middle classes in urban India. The traders of drugs in the bazaars continued to supply consumers with their drugs of widely varying potency. However, since everyone concerned had internalised the tropes of purity/impurity or scientific/unscientific indicators for drugs, a formal Indian pharmacopeia could not be published until after independence. Instead, the conflicts over the legitimacy of Indigenous medicine were played out in their institution-building; the new Ayurveda or Unani colleges, industrial manufacture of Indigenous medicine, and in the market itself. In the following chapters, we will examine the dualities of purity and adulteration in the crowded medical marketplace of colonial India and the place of 'Indigenous' drugs at their institutional sites. In the next chapter, we will examine how the colonial government itself acted as a major producer and distributor of drugs in India, especially during the two world wars.

Conclusion

The impossibility of the Indian pharmacopeia reflected the medical culture of India in the late nineteenth and early twentieth century. The demand for the publication of a formal Indian pharmacopeia was engendered by multiple concerns. These were commercial and ideological, representing the real and symbolic objectives of substituting cheaper alternatives for expensive, imported drugs; achieving standardisation in the potency of clearly identified drugs and consequently the greater availability of a number of drugs for treatment; and the formal confirmation of the place and significance of Indian drugs internationally. Finally, the establishment of an Indian pharmacopeia represented the status of India as a site of enlightened scientific and medical praxis. The commercial imperatives for an Indian pharmacopeia were clear; it would have strengthened the domestic medical market. It was an emotive issue for nationalist politics that was steeped in the politics of economic and cultural nationalism. A formal Indian pharmacopeia would have validated Indigenous medical systems to a significant extent, enriching prevalent narratives of the value of Indigenous, pre-colonial episteme. Yet, it was the very prolificacy of drugs and the resultant uncertainty about identifying their potency that rendered the task of formulating an Indian pharmacopeia both urgent and difficult. A colonial government, which depended on manufactured drugs from its metropolitan centres, would not summon enthusiasm for the project except during the two world wars when the imports had to be stopped. Therefore, the publication of the Indian pharmacopeia had to await the establishment of the new nation-state.

In 1955, when the Indian pharmacopeia was finally published, the landscape of drug use was transformed through the use of sulphonamides, synthetic anti-malarial drugs, and antibiotics, which process was further hastened by the radical outcomes achieved in military medicine during the Second World War.[67] The newly emergent postcolonial nation under Nehru was far more focussed on acquiring access to technology and infrastructure for the manufacture of sulpha drugs and antibiotics. In 1955, the official Indian pharmacopeia was published to validate and emphasise the new nation-state's authority and its political identity, now distinct from the British Empire. When finally published, the official Indian Pharmacopeia sabotaged its raison d'être, dreamed of initially by its colonial advocates, and instead of utilising Indian drugs, relegated these to a marginal status.

4

The Promises and Forfeiture of Import Substitution

While the realisation of the dream of an Indian pharmacopeia remained elusive in colonial India, Indian drugs, or indeed, Indigenous systems of medicine continued to flourish in markets, therapeutic practices, and medical literature. Indian drugs were processed and marketed within the subcontinent and globally. Meanwhile, in the emergent public sphere, debates on public health, the legitimacy of Indigenous epistemology including its medicine, and the nature of the ideal masculine/feminine Indian bodies and how these could be achieved, were numerous and voluble.[1] The scholarly consensus is that Ayurveda, in particular, was legitimised through the reinforcement of Sanskrit textual evidence.[2] The Unani system experienced this too, and its orthodox elements were relatively marginalised in public discourse.[3] Its practitioners, even among long-established families, were mostly willing to consider the 'unity' of Tibb with modern Western medical techniques and to institutionalise their pedagogy.[4] In colonial India, medical praxis was dynamic among practitioners of Indigenous and Western medicine.[5]

There was, however, one context that ran as a common thread: the availability of medicines to the dispenser and the medical consumer. Much of the discourse and praxis of 'harmony' between Indigenous and Western medical systems occurred in the historical context of the availability or the scarcity of medicines and therapies. This chapter will examine the activities of the Government Medical Store (GMS), which was controlled by the Indian army and remained the principal distributor of medicines, both imported and of its own manufacture, to civil hospitals, and was in charge of the cultivation of new drugs. The GMS is significant because it was the largest single producer, importer, and distributor of medical therapies in colonial India. Therefore, it was at the centre of debates on government policy and Indian industrialization in the pharmaceutical industry in nationalist discourse.

Historians have intensely debated colonial industrialization. Scholars have pointed out how British capital dominated Indian industrialization in the tea, jute, coffee, and leather goods sectors.[6] Others have pointed out how Indigenous trading firms shifted their capital from trade to industry in several sectors – most importantly in textiles, sugar, cement, and paper – between the two world wars and show how the model of agency firms leached profits and slowed down innovation within British-Indian industry.[7] Lately, T. Roy has argued that the incorporation of the Indian economy within the global commercial system and the investments in infrastructure and governance were representative of how British policies enabled the Indian economy towards growth in the twentieth century.[8] The new economic history has directed attention towards small-scale industry and artisan trades and highlighted the histories of smaller towns and their industrial units.[9] Nonetheless. large-scale industrial units in critical sectors such as steel, hydraulic power, machine tools, and heavy chemicals only gained momentum with strong state support and protectionism in Nehruvian India, although the ideology of this model of development dominated Indian nationalist discourse by the 1940s.[10]

The pharmaceutical manufacturing industry was located somewhere in the middle of this spectrum. Several categories of medicines could be manufactured with the aid of only a copy of the BP, a skilled chemist, a small distilling plant, and a few chemicals and raw drugs, as P.C. Ray had proven in the early 1890s.[11] And indeed, many smaller drug manufacturers who produced a handful of proprietary medicines in the form of pills and powders and a few galenicals did so with similarly rudimentary infrastructure even in the 1930s.[12] Yet for an economically viable concern it was vital to scale up the volume of production and invest in researching new drugs. As the examples of ACWL and BCPW have demonstrated, state support in the form of testing laboratories, tariff and railway freight concessions, and access to new drugs and distribution networks were fundamental to the continued success of the firms.[13] These conditions were all met in British India by the government's own manufacturing unit, the GMS.

The Government Medical Store and the Problem of Substitution

The GMS was established in 1858 and was a remnant of the East India Company's military medical stores establishment. 'Medical stores' at Bombay, Madras, Calcutta, Lahore, and Rangoon served as collection points for raw drugs and warehouses for storing imported drugs for distribution; the Bombay and Madras stores produced the most therapeutic products. From the mid-nineteenth century, the government established and aided hospitals in the metropolis and planned for an extended subscription-based dispensary in provincial districts in British India.[14] In the late nineteenth century, the government encouraged the proliferation of charitable hospitals and dispensaries in the provincial districts (rather than establish government hospitals as in the metropolises) and supplied these medicines from the GMS, extending its role in the institutional expansion of Western medicine.

Historians have argued that nationalist discourse and the Swadeshi cause occasioned the expansion of the medicinal and chemical industry at the turn of the century.[15] The scholarly consensus is that import substitution played a dominant role in government support to Indian industry after the First World War. As far as pharmaceutical commodities were concerned, however, import substitution was not only a nationalist cause, nor was it merely a geopolitical response to imperial rivalries between the two world wars. From the 1870s, the possibilities of even partially substituting therapeutic substances imported from abroad entranced, albeit intermittently, officials in Whitehall and Simla who were charged with restricting the Government of India's expenditure. Therefore, while the government encouraged the use of hospitals and dispensaries, it simultaneously promoted the sale of medicines supplied by the GMS to these hospitals. An overwhelming proportion of these were rudimentary therapies for commonly occurring diseases in the region; quinine for malaria, the ubiquitous cholera pills and chiretta, an Indigenous drug used for dysentery and diarrhoea.[16] In 1872, for instance, the Bengal government reported that it was 'glad to observe that the total value of medicines sold … had improved in the late 1871'. The provincial government rued at the same time that, 'the increase is solely due to the large sales of quinine. The sale of jalap, cheyretta, and cholera pills has not improved'.[17]

As the government expected to extend the establishment and use of mofussil dispensaries and Western medicine, it also explored the possibilities of processing as many drugs as possible from the raw materials already available in India. The proliferation of the manufacture of processed Western medical therapies occurred first through the government's own requirements and priorities. In 1876, the Government of India instituted an enquiry committee to find out how the GMS could reduce its expenditure on medicines and allied commodities through the greater use of local drugs and raw materials processed within its own workshops in Bombay or Madras. The committee's findings were instructive. The GMS imported items in bulk like lime juice and oils when these could be replaced with easily processed local products. The committee was appalled to find out that:

> Indeed there is good reason for believing that a considerable portion of the olive oil of commerce is but the Jinjili or ground nut oils of India, for, besides large exports of both oils to Europe, several thousand tons of the sesamum seed and ground nuts ... are exported annually from the south of India to France, where the oil is expressed and finds its way into the market as olive oil ... there would have been a considerable saving in Bengal using the native oil.[18]

The report revealed that botanical materials that were abundantly available in one part of the subcontinent were being exported abroad and the same or similar products were being imported at a much greater cost in a different part:

> 138 lbs. of *Cantharides* were shipped to Bombay in 1872-74 at 7s. 6d. per lb ... From Madras, it is reported that the *Mylabris cichorii*, or Teline fly, is used as a substitute for *Cantharides* ... During the years of which the lists are given, 336 lbs. appear to have been issued from the stores ... It seems desirable that Bombay Medical Stores should procure the *Mylabris* either from Madras or Calcutta.[19]

This was not unique to drugs; products used widely in medicine such as cod liver oil were available cheaply in Madras and simultaneously imported at more than four times the cost in Bombay. Moreover, Bombay itself exported thousands of tons of fish oil to England and the committee's report mused that 'it is more than probable that a portion of this finds its way into the cod liver oil of commerce'.[20] A great many of the expensive imports of the GMS from Britain could be substituted by having each of the presidency Medical Stores share the products and substitutions from their respective local markets. The substitutions offered were standard ones used widely within India (and in the international drug markets) – cassia bark for cinnamon; chiretta for squill pills, and gingelley oil for the imported olive oil used in liniments. Others were expensive imports into one presidency capital where local markets in any of the others provided the same ingredients at lower prices, such as the extract of colocynth. The committee identified twenty-three such drugs or botanical materials that could be either procured or their local substitutes obtained without taking recourse to expensive imported drugs. Given that an average of 400 drugs were listed in the Indian materia medica at this time and at least fifty or sixty were used extensively, this was a miniscule list. In addition, there were recommendations for the GMS to extend its own pharmaceutical operations and the manufacture of chemicals essential to drug manufacturing, for instance, sulphuric acid, nitric and hydrochloric acids, ether, and spirit of ammonia. There were some private British-Indian manufacturers of chemicals in Bombay and Calcutta who cost the GMS far less than the imported acids, but the relative ease and economy of manufacture within the GMS would have tempted the suggestion to manufacture these within the GMS factories.

Moreover, the committee (advised by J.D. Hooker, the renowned botanist and the director of Kew Garden) suggested cultivating drugs in government plantations for final processing by the GMS. At this time, government plantations in the Madras presidency were beginning to produce cinchona, although these turned out to be an inferior variety to the more potent Javanese varieties.[21]

J.D. Hooker, who had conducted botanical expeditions (and imperial adventure) in the eastern Himalayas and was familiar with Indian conditions, suggested 'that some medicinal plants in constant use grow luxuriantly in certain parts of India ... others would thrive with very slight care.[22] He named twenty-two drugs that were widely known and used and could be cultivated in the various Indian conditions. These included artemisia, belladonna,

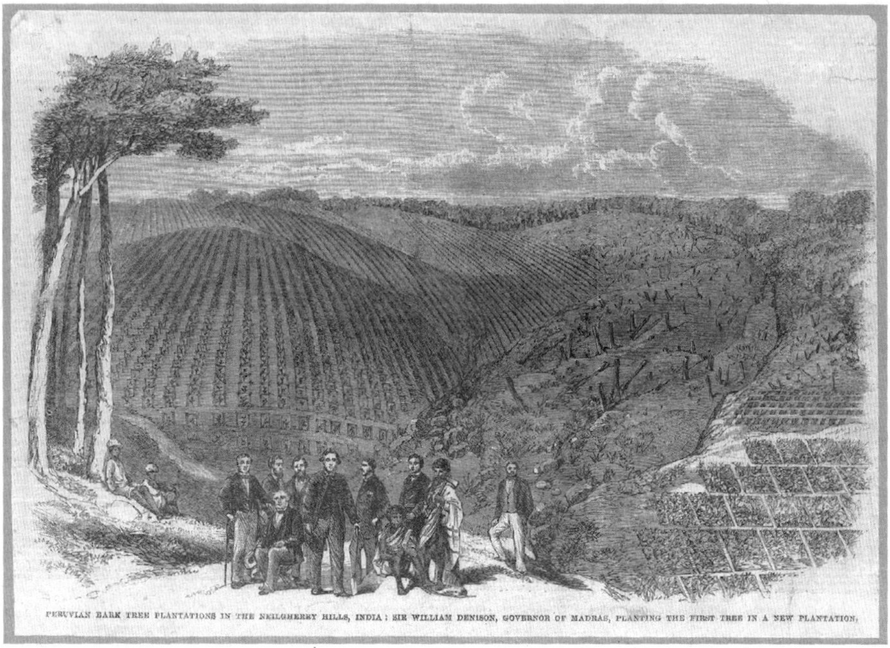
PERUVIAN BARK TREE PLANTATIONS IN THE NEILGHERRY HILLS, INDIA: SIR WILLIAM DENISON, GOVERNOR OF MADRAS, PLANTING THE FIRST TREE IN A NEW PLANTATION.

Figure 4.1 Sir W. Denison and others planting the first cinchona trees in the Nilgiris, c.1862

digitalis, gentian, and ipecacuanha; all of which were well-known drugs and were cultivated in India to varying degrees in succeeding decades.

However, affable suggestions to extend and diversify the capacity and variety of drugs within India did little to change the minds of the IMS officials in charge of the GMS. Never known for its radical approach, the IMS continued to rely on British manufacturers. Moreover, the report's recommendations drew retaliation from British drug manufacturing and exporting interests. The Society of Apothecaries was the principal beneficiary of the expensive imports to India. The Society had enjoyed the lucrative monopoly of supplying all drugs to the East India Company from 1766 until 1858 and continued to supply a substantial proportion of the Indian army's medical supplies after the takeover by the Crown. The Society also enjoyed the monopoly of supply to the Navy until 1805 and continued to supply the Navy after the monopoly ceased. Its profit margins were substantial. A pamphlet in 1747 suggested that it was as much as 60 per cent.[23] Scholars suggest that the Society's reputation for excellent quality enabled it to sustain very high prices.[24] Possibly the close and intertwined commercial and social networks between the two institutions further enabled the monopoly.

When the Society's monopoly of supplies was terminated by the EIC, the Secretary of State for India's office took to taking out tenders annually for the supply of all drugs to India. These tenders were won by large establishments in London (e.g., the firms of Howard and Sons and British Drug House) as well as the Society of Apothecaries. In 1869, for instance, almost all imported drugs from Britain in all three presidencies were ordered from the Society.[25] Therefore, the attention to lower costs for drugs on the Government of India's part served to direct the government's purchases to suppliers within Britain itself, displacing the old monopoly. In 1875, the Society, having lost out on tenders to other British firms, pointed out to the Governor General's office in India that 'The prices which are quoted in what are called trade lists are such could not possibly procure medicines suitable for the public service in India, and the Society consider that no just comparison can be made of their medicines with such lists'.[26] The Society remained 'anxious to maintain the good understanding which has for so many years existed between them and the GOI [Government of India]', but direct orders from the Government of India to the Society of Apothecaries ceased altogether in 1882. However, almost all of the GMS's requisitions continued to be made from Britain where their tenders were advertised.[27]

Although the GMS committee's report advised, as much as possible, for government-controlled cultivation and production of drugs through the replacement or substitution of locally available bazaar medicines, there was little expectation that these suggestions would be met substantially. Instead, the report limited the extent of requests any hospital could make to the GMS; indents could only be submitted once annually and itemised minutely, including in-advance provisioning budgeting for any epidemic.[29] The army hospitals were allowed to buy some bazaar medicines locally in emergencies, but the amount to be spent on these was strictly curtailed too. As a retired army official recounted at the turn of the century:

> The supply of drugs [in native army hospitals] is not nearly so good as In station-hospitals, [British hospitals] whilst the supplies of instruments and surgical dressings is meagre in the extreme. If the doctor wants a remedy not allowed according to the 'Scale of Drugs', he must either purchase it himself or induce the Colonel to obtain it out of some regimental fund.[30]

The report's recommendations were mostly ignored in official policy. However, the significance of the report is that it identified and articulated concerns that would resonate within the medical and official establishment in India for the next seventy-odd years. The use of local raw drugs, extending production in manufacturing workshops of the GMS, cultivating non-native drugs within government plantations, and collating and popularizing a functional Indian pharmacopeia remained the critical aspects of making medicines in colonial India. Government policy and implementation meandered their way through most of the recommendations. Government cinchona plantations were established and maintained in the Nilgiris and the Darjeeling hills from the 1880s and the cinchona was processed within the GMS, although these did not come close to meeting the demands for quinine in colonial India. The government botanical gardens experimented with cultivating several of the twenty-two drugs that the committee had suggested on advice from J.D. Hooker. But none were produced in the quantities or quality that were adequate for the supply to Indian hospitals and dispensaries.

The Expansion and the Limits of the GMS

GMS's extension of services to civilian medical institutions occurred because the military managed civil government medical services. At first, the Medical Stores in Bombay, Calcutta, Madras, and Lahore were managed within the presidency but starting in 1894, they were re-organised and controlled centrally from the DGIMS's office. With the recommendation for centralisation of procurement in 1875, the limited purchase of Indigenous drugs at the local market by officials in charge of even non-governmental, civil hospitals was severely curtailed. In 1900, the principal of the Bombay Veterinary College had to seek permission for the sanction of drugs worth a relatively insignificant sum of Rs 37.50/- and explain that 'that the purchase was made from the local market under unavoidable circumstances'.[31] This loss of autonomy for local hospitals and military regiments to buy directly from their bazaars except in absolute emergencies identified the GMS as the central point of production and also distribution. The requisitions were made by the DGIMS's office in consultation with the Medical Storekeepers of the presidency capitals, who were all British IMS officials. The restriction on buying bazaar medicines by any hospital increased the GMS's expenses for the distribution of the drugs. The ambition of import substitution of non-Indigenous (and even Indigenous) drugs was eclipsed and the GMS continued the expensive import of most drugs. The DGIMS, F.N. Macnamara, who was one of the three members of the special committee who wrote the report of 1875, went to the extent of expressing his regrets that he could not order medicines in bulk from the Society of Apothecaries, whose quality of goods he believed were incomparable. Instead, the DGIMS's office invited tenders from 'established' London-based manufacturers. These comprised a handful of firms such as Messrs Howard and Sons and Messrs Savour and Moore. By the turn of the century, the best-known UK-based manufacturers were lobbying hard to keep their lucrative orders from the Government of India for the GMS. In 1902, for instance, B.W. & Co. instructed their agent in Bombay to:

> Arrange with reliable and safe person at Simla to inform us at once should it be necessary for firm's representative to be present on Govt matters during your absence we must be quite certain our interest will not be endangered by neglect.
>
> ... we are anxious for you to make such arrangements as may be necessary to ensure our being informed should any special crisis in connection with the supply of Tabloid and Soloid products to the Indian Government.[32]

In the early 1900s, the GMS was still extensively importing drugs and processed therapeutic products from British firms, although it had expanded its own manufactures. The monopoly of supply from the Society of Apothecaries had disappeared but imports were limited to a few manufacturing firms in London that aggressively pursued the GMS's custom. The GMS stopped providing medicines freely or at cost to government hospitals in 1891 under the advice of the military medical office.[33] At this time, the GMS derived substantial profits from its distribution to civil hospitals, non-government dispensaries, and hospitals. Its profits from the sale of medicines to these institutions subsidised the military medical expenses of the army in India. In 1906, for instance, the Military Finance Department ordered that the *ganja* (cannabis indica) supplied to the GMS in Madras would be free of cost and from excise duty, but that 'an extra-department charge of 10 per cent will be levied when the depot issues it or articles containing it to non-Government institutions, the amount so realised being treated as receipts in the Military Accounts'.[34]

Medicines and the Military-Commercial Enterprise

While import substitution was a nationalist aspiration in political rhetoric after the First World War, substitution was on the government's agenda too, though less visibly than in its nationalist form, as a cost-cutting measure from the 1900s. The GMS was required to provide the army hospitals with free pharmaceutical products; it financed these as well as turned a net profit on its sales to local, civil, and voluntary hospitals and dispensaries. With financial pressure from the military authorities on the GMS to ensure profitability from its sales and the concomitant great expansion in voluntary hospitals and dispensaries from the late nineteenth century, the financial gains were substantial. The DGIMS reported that, except for Bombay and Lahore, the three other GMS made profits by selling their products to civil institutions. The DGIMS pointed out that the profits generated by the sale to non-government civil institutions by the GMS were critical to the military medical department:

> [The GMS] supplies some Native States and a very large number of institutions which are maintained by Municipalities, Local Boards, etc … The question of policy involved is one that cannot, with propriety, discussed here; but it may be stated that, if the custom of Civil-Local Institutions were withdrawn the efficiency of the (Medical) Department would be greatly impaired, and a heavy burden would be thrown on the Military Budget.[35]

Until the First World War, when imports stopped almost completely, the GMS had two objectives: to supply high-quality therapeutic commodities to the military medical establishments in the Indian army; and to encourage the institutionalisation of the hospital system through the sale of medicines to civil institutions in British India and the princely states. The GMS was a complex institution; the five medical stores did not all manufacture therapeutic products or process drugs. The Bombay and the Madras stores' 'workshops' (in effect they were factories) manufactured finished therapeutic products. The Calcutta store collected botanical drug supplies and processed a few therapeutic products as well as acted as a warehouse and distributing centre in eastern India. The Lahore and Rangoon branches were principally warehouses and distribution centres for the military and civil institutions in their respective regions. In 1909, the manufactures of the GMS included more than 265 pharmaceutical products including galenicals, pills, powders, ointments and gels, surgical bandages, extracts, and essential oils.[36] Excepting branded proprietary medicines, this was the range of therapies manufactured by several other firms at the time, including the British-owned and Indian manufacturer/distributors like Stanistreet, Smith and Co. or Treacher and Co., N. Powell and Co., or the ACWL and the BCPW. The difference was in the scale of the manufactures. The GMS was larger than any one private manufacturer; in 1909/10, the Madras factory produced 60,000 lb. of tinctures. The GMS's products included therapies containing opium that was processed at the government opium factory at Ghazipur and Patna. Unsurprisingly, the largest proportion of the pharmaceutical production was the manufacture of quinine processed from the Government cinchona plantations in the Nilgiris and the Darjeeling hills; in 1909/10, these amounted to more than seven million tablets and pills. This represented an enormously increased production by the GMS factories; in the previous year, their production of quinine tablets was less than two million.[37]

This prodigious increase in production served to utilise locally grown raw drugs. A substantial proportion of these comprised the produce from government plantations and botanical gardens, as well as the monopolistic access to all legally cultivated poppies in British India. The cultivation, processing, sale, and use of opium and its derivatives were tightly controlled under a monopoly that was first imposed by the EIC in eighteenth-century Bengal.[38] Opium and its derivatives were subject to excise duties. The GMS enjoyed the first use of opium in its factories without having to pay any excise duties, providing a point of resentment to local manufacturers. What the GMS could not use of the raw opium was exported abroad or sold to carefully vetted manufacturing firms in India. By the time the GMS expanded its production in the early 1900s, the sale of (legal) opium had declined substantially from the 1870s. Nonetheless, morphine, codeine, and opium-laced proprietary medicines and other clinical products continued to be available in substantial quantities in the medical market, of which the highest volume was produced in the GMS.

Therefore, the substitution of expensive imported drugs by locally manufactured products and the concomitant expansion of the GMS before the First World War, while significant, were essentially selective. Most of its production involved two or three locally produced drugs. Nonetheless, their advantages in access to technical expertise, labour, and other infrastructure through the Indian army put them in an advantageous position vis-à-vis competing private firms in Calcutta and Bombay. The GMS administration was acutely aware of the competition from private trade. The DGIMS declared in 1910–11:

> There is no tendency among Local Governments to give up dealing with the Medical Store Department. On the contrary, the administration of the NWFP, having withdrawn its custom and obtained supplies from the trade, has now recommenced dealing with the Lahore Depot.[39]

The GMS had the advantage of large-scale production (especially of quinine) and base chemicals for pharmaceuticals, such as sulphuric and hydrochloric acids. It had ready access to medical expertise from armed forces personnel, priority access to raw drugs within India, and was afforded government protection with customs duties and railway freight charges. These enabled it to sustain a prized reputation for quality pharmaceutical products made with B.P. specifications and sustained a healthy profit for the military medical department *after* having supplied the military with its own requirements. Its relatively high prices compared to private firms in the bazaar were noticed by the urban Indian public.[40]

Nonetheless, the GMS's productions were limited compared to the more expensive pharmaceutical commodities bought from 'home', i.e., from Britain. A part of the GMS's costs of drugs from 'home' was for raw drugs or essential chemicals that were used to process local Indian drugs, but most were finished goods, including compressed pills and tabloids. In 1909/10, for instance, the GMS's expenditure on 'home' products was substantially greater than the previous year's but authorities were still confident that, although 'the home expenditure rose from, roughly, 6.57 to 10.23 lakhs; and this increase...will no doubt be followed by a proportionate increase in receipts' in the next financial year.[41] Yet, even with the heavier spend on commodities from 'home' and without the benefit of the profits that were expected to accrue from these, in 1909/10 the receipts from its sales amounted to Rs 12,88,202, with a profit of Rs 1,90,746.[42]

The profits were higher in some presidencies than in others. These were calculated after the military units assigned in the respective regions had been served with pharmaceutical and other medical products at no cost. Generally, the Calcutta, Madras, and Burma medical stores turned out higher profits than their counterparts in Lahore and Bombay because they could supply a smaller quantity of medical products to the lucrative civil institutions after supplying to the higher numbers of military units stationed in their respective regions.[43]

As table 4.1 shows, the number of civil institutions supplied by the GMS increased steadily until the First World War. These included government-aided hospitals (civil institutions) but also smaller charitable municipal and local hospitals and dispensaries and supplies to similar institutions within the princely states. This was representative of the broader expansion of the dispensary and hospital system in the Indian subcontinent and the corresponding rise in the demand for therapeutic products within the hospital system. The number of local and civic bodies and princely states supplied with GMS's pharmaceutical products points to the near monopoly of the GMS.

The GMS, by far the largest supplier of pharmaceutical and therapeutic products in India, operated within a classically colonial relationship with British medicine; it exported raw drugs in bulk and imported finished pharmaceutical products that it re-distributed to the Indian army and sold to civil institutions at profit. The profits from the transactions subsidised medicines and equipment provided to the Indian army with the fiscal burden of the army's medical needs falling on the civil and charitable hospitals. In 1912, the Finance Department of the GOI provided figures that demonstrated

Table 4.1
Institutions supplied by the Medical Store: 1909/10–1912/13

Year	*Military*	*Civil*	*Civic & local bodies*	*Native states*	*RIN (Royal Navy)*	*RIM (Royal Marine)*	*Unclassified (opium only)*	*Total*
1909/10	470	1524	528	102	10	17	324	2975
1910/11	614	1279	880	89	09	17	317	3205
1911/12	720	1396	868	103	08	17	295	3407
1912/13	892	1489	902	094	08	14	239	3638

Source: GMS Annual Reports for relevant years, IOR/APAC.

Table 4.2
Expenditure and income from medicine and allied products by the GMS 1895/96–1912/13

	Products from 'home' (pound sterling)	*Products from India (pound sterling)*	*Total (pound sterling)*
1895–96 to 1899–1900			
Average expenditure	23,356	35,061	58,417
Average receipts from sale	20,842	19,230	40,072
Average net expenditure	2,514	15,831	18,345
1905–06 to 1908–09			
Average expenditure	47,785	47,331	95,116
Average receipts	30,706	29,052	59,758
Average net expenditure	17,079	18,279	35,358
1909–10 to 1912–13			
Average expenditure	88,195	47,942	136,137
Average receipts	47,654	35,337	82,991
Average net expenditure	40,541	12,695	53,146

Source: Memo on the course of Military expenditure 1898–99 to 1912–3, Appendix 5, L/MIL/17/5/1903/APAC/BL.

that the GMS subsidised most of the Indian army's medical expenses in spite of the increase in costs through an expansion in the supply to civil institutions in the previous three decades: 'The sales ... civil institutions] are rapidly increasing ... the true cost [to military expense] is diminished by the profit on sales'.[44] It also clarified that although medical expenses had increased in the previous two decades, most of the 'real' rise in expenses had been absorbed by the sale of medicines and in the much lower sickness levels in the Indian army.[45]

Table 4.2 demonstrates year-on-year increases in the expenditure on medicines imported from 'home', with the costs almost doubling every five years. Meanwhile, the GMS's spending on products from India remained fairly constant. Therefore, the exhortations to generate import substitution by the government in India were to maintain lower costs and subsidise the Indian army through the GMS. The GMS did not expand its production of processed therapeutic commodities in the Indian medical market, although it had clear advantages over local manufacturers. This kept the cost of supplies to the Indian army high. It also reduced the range and quantity of therapeutic commodities available to the Indian medical consumer. And it kept the Indian army and the public dependent on imports from the UK. All of these were to be shaken by the First World War.

The War and the Search for Substitutes: Local Production with Indigenous Drugs

The First World War brought the local production of medicines into the public eye. India's contribution to the war effort included a multitude of human, animal, and material resources. The dependence on Britain for most imports of manufactured goods highlighted the Indian army's and the RAMC's vulnerabilities. The stimulus for manufacture came from the munitions board and included the expansion of existing capacities, organisation of known agricultural resources for industrial production, and finally, the 'search for substitutes'.[46] These included the supply of khakis and leather for uniforms; steel from the newly established Tata Iron and Steel Works; and medicine, surgical materials, bandages, ointments, antiseptic agents, acids, and glass for phials, etc.

Once the imports from Europe and the USA stopped, the siphoning of available resources in the subcontinent for the British and Indian armies generated great scarcity in the open market. Not just the consuming public; medical practitioners voiced their anger and helplessness at the situation and the clamour for government support for Indigenous medicine in India grew louder.

Indeed, the period between the wars saw an unprecedented rise in Indian manufacturing industries including steel and machine tools, chemicals, glass, and cement, as well as consumer items like matches, electric bulbs, and umbrellas, in addition to the more traditional textile, leather, and jute industries. The GOI commissioned an Indian Industrial Committee in 1916, chaired by T.H. Holland to review and suggest ways of establishing an industrial base in India. This briefly created a common aim between official and nationalist discourse in post-WWI India. The Indian Industrial Commission (Holland Report) in 1918 recognised the vital significance of chemical industries in British India – munitions and medicines, two essential components of fighting wars depended on these.[47] T.H. Holland was also the chair of the munitions board in India so it was clear that the impetus for industrialization came from war-based necessities.[48] It also famously recommended an all-India Chemical Service to encourage and consolidate expertise in chemical sciences, without which, it declared, industrialization would not be possible.[49] As historians have pointed out, the Commission's report and its strong advice for the government to support a plan of industrialization for India was ignored, although most provincial governments set up a department of industry and made a few scattered attempts at establishing technological research centres to aid industry.[50] Individual officials like Holland or D.K. Chadwick, who offered evidence and argument for these, were ineffective in influencing policy.[51]

Once the war was over, the Munitions Board showed little interest in extending the capacity of the GMS or in investing in technological expertise. An IMS committee was appointed to oversee the transfer of the department of health from central to provincial governments under new political reforms. This committee clarified that the government did not envisage any need for the GMS to extend its operations to supply medicines and therapeutic products to the proliferating number of civil and local hospitals in British India: 'The Committee consider that the Medical Stores Department has at present as much work as can be carried out without considerable expansion … they do not think it advisable to press for any extension'.[52] The immediacy of import substitution on the part of the GMS faded after the war. Nor was the GMS an exception here; the manufactures of the ordinance factories of the government suffered a similar fate of stalled expansion and inferior technology that could not support new manufactures.[53]

The GMS itself, as the principal manufacturer or importer of drugs and therapies, did not undergo fundamental policy changes or hugely expand either cultivation or manufacture of drugs locally. Nonetheless, there was enough anxiety in the government about the dependence of the Indian army on imports and the crises that might ensue as consequence. The war had, after all, exposed the vulnerability of the Indian army in its dependence on imports of even basic pharmaceutical and surgical products. But both the government's and medical officials' focus remained on identifying which new drugs could be cultivated and how to isolate the active principles of known Indigenous drugs. There was little focus on their manufacture by the GMS. Meanwhile, the disastrous Mesopotamian campaign in the First World War, which involved the Indian army and represented catastrophic errors in the logistics and quality of medical supplies for the Indian army, generated public fury in Britain and dismay in official circles in India.[54] Several established pharmaceutical firms, such as Smith, Stanistreet, and Co., Bathgate and Co., B.K. Paul and Co., continued to supply raw drugs as well as finished medical preparations to the GMS as well as to firms in London, Glasgow, Hong Kong, Manila, New York, Paris, and Australia throughout the war.[55] Several firms based in Bombay and Karachi, such as Messrs D.P. Ghandy and Co., Messrs Narottam Girdhar and Co., and J.F. Madan and Co., shipped drugs and medicines directly to Basra during the war.[56] Therefore, the drugs that would have been available in the private market were diverted to the war effort by the government as well as by private traders and manufacturers at the same time as stopping the import of therapeutic commodities from Britain.

The scarcity of imported drugs and medicines during the war added to the existing problem of dilution or adulteration of drugs. Moffusil medical men reported that the quinine tablets available in the districts, which tended to be adulterated before the war, had gotten worse after a substantial rise in prices during the war: 'This indiscriminate adulteration is going on in a larger scale'.[57] The shortages and price rise in all drugs also facilitated an expansion in the scale and variety of drugs under manufacture by local British and Indian manufacturers. Smith, Stanistreet and Co. built a new factory and moved to new offices in Calcutta to accommodate their extended operations. They also increased their consumption of raw drugs within India and exported finished products like thymol to London.[58] Several new firms manufacturing drugs and medicines, both 'Ayurvedic' and Western, as well as firms manufacturing sera and vaccines, tried to fill the gap from the diversion of drugs, sera and vaccines to the war effort. This was helped by scientific and technical expertise available through university-educated chemists as well as the more traditional medical practitioners. For instance, the Bengal Immunity Company (established 1919), a joint venture of P.C. Ray and a few Indian physicians employed at Calcutta hospitals began to manufacture vaccines and sera, hitherto only produced by the government research institute at Kasauli and the Haffkine Institute in Bombay. Correspondingly, the demand for local, cheaper alternatives to expensive, imported foreign drugs occasioned the rise of several manufacturing firms especially in Bombay and Calcutta, many venturing into the new profitable business for the first time. As the author of *Commercial Drugs of India,* a manual for new entrepreneurs pointed out, his book was:

> intended not so much for the medical practitioner ... as for the business man. While stating the medicinal and other economic uses of plants in a brief way, this book aims at placing at the disposal of the drug grower, collector or dealer all available information regarding the sources, methods of collection, cultivation and marketing of Indian drugs or drugs that may be grown in India ... The new spirit of industrial revival which is manifest all over the country has not and will not leave the drug industry unaffected. The so-called drugs, it should be noted, are not used for medicinal purposes only. The same plant which yields a drug may be equally or more valuable as a dye or tan stuff, perfumery ingredient, spice or food-stuff.[59]

In the final instance, medical and official discourse, as well as commercial opinion in British firms, focussed on the cultivation of drugs and the 'scientific study' of Indigenous drugs rather than on the manufacture of finished goods that might compete with British imports.[60] Indian medical practitioners recognised that Indigenous drugs would be invaluable and cheaper than imported material if manufactured within India. To them, the prospect of collaboration and cooperation between the practitioners of Western medicine and Indigenous systems seemed possible, even a necessity. Sir Nil Ratan Sircar, the President of the All-India Medical Conference, an association of Indian medical practitioners, strongly advocated for the introduction of Indian therapeutics and the study of Indian drugs in 1919.

Medical Discourse and Local Drugs for Local Treatments

The nationalist and medical discourse moved closer to praxis in the market facilitated by the scarcity of drugs in the open market during the First World War.[61] The market, as we have seen, was heterogeneous and accommodating of eclectic medical praxis. The BCPW and ACWL, the premier scientific pharmaceutical companies at this time, both specialised in Indigenous and Western therapies. So did a host of other British-Indian manufacturers, including Smith, Stanistreet and Co., which like many other manufacturers had made impressive gains during the war.[62] At this juncture it seemed feasible to adapt Western medicine to Indian drugs, although there was a need to verify their active principles. As a medical official at the Madras General Hospital pointed out in 1918:

> I feel unable to comprehend why one should not try to understand the actions of simpler drugs as Carminative, Aromatic stimulants, laxatives, etc. as also the therapeutical uses of drugs, familiar to us, i.e., drugs common to both the Indigenous and our own Pharmacopoeia. You can leave the Professor to find out what active principles are contained in the different drugs and to which of them their actions are due. But I think that if the drugs are really of any value, you may preferably make use of them instead of the dearer and more inaccessible foreign drugs … The invaluable use of an acquaintance with the Indigenous drug, can best be realised in the country. The drug will not only be very cheap but you can get it at a moment's notice from any nook and corner of the country.[63]

The Indigenous pharmaceutical manufacturers such as Gopalacharu, Zandu, Dabur, and Hamdard had made substantial gains through their clever and extensive advertising in the regional and English presses.[64] In 1925, the Ayurvedic medicines firm in Bombay, ZPL (established 1910), moved to new and larger premises and celebrated a remarkable rise in its sales from Rs 7,638 in 1910 to Rs 21,0743 in 1924. This trend in medical discourse strengthened the case for import substitution. The prevalent discourse of tropical drugs for tropical bodies and, indeed, the reiteration of these in new diagnoses and nomenclatures of 'tropical neurasthenia' and 'tropical diabetes' along with the persistence of older nomenclature such as 'tropical dysentery' reinforced the geography/climate/race tropes in the occurrence of disease.[65] Even the *IMG*, the official voice of the IMS, speculated that the Western medical practitioner in India would experience a different set of diseases and come across a few drugs that would be quite distinct from any clinical education or experience in Britain.[66]

Moreover, the deterioration of imported drugs in the Indian climate became an issue between the wars when new research enabled transnational companies to produce hormonal drugs (for diabetes and heart disease, for instance) and vitamins that were highly sensitive to climate and storage conditions. As Major R.N. Chopra, IMS, of Calcutta School of Tropical Medicine declared in his presidential address to the Medical and Veterinary Research section of the Indian Science Congress at Lahore in 1927:

> With regard to the imported drugs, which form by far the largest proportion of drugs used in India, most of them are manufactured by reputed firms who employ a competent staff of chemists and pharmacologists to standardise them. The climatic conditions however, in this country have to be taken into consideration. A few years ago my laboratory tested nearly a hundred preparations of digitalis made by reputed firms and found that most of these had deteriorated to the extent of 30 to 40 per cent within a few months of their arrival in India. Some drugs such as thyroid extract, etc are similarly affected. Several batches of old tablets of pituitrin and adrenalin, and some containing potent alkaloids which we tested had appreciably deteriorated in quality. The keeping properties of organical arsenicals, and a number of other potent remedies, when exposed to tropical climates, still remain to be worked out.[67]

At this time, therefore, import substitution, as well as the regular use of Indigenous drugs by practitioners of all systems that was a feature of medical praxis in India, achieved a great degree of legitimacy in official and medical discourse. However, this was not an endorsement of Indigenous medicine or its practitioners. This was a continuation of the nineteenth-century expediency of using bazaar medicines. It also validated transnational pharmaceutical firms using Indigenous drugs for their own patents. Items like 'chiretta', for instance, were routinely used and Moore's medical handbook, the eighth edition of which was published in 1916, prescribed Indigenous drugs like datura, jambul, and neem in its formularies.[68] Indigenous drugs, like chaulmugra oil, were manufactured by all reputable drug companies and entered the medical lexicon of all practitioners in India, both Western and Indigenous, including homeopathic practitioners.[69] By 1909, F. Bayer had received a patent for their mixture of chaulmugra oil.[70] Meanwhile, Dr Bose's Laboratory, a manufacturing pharmacy set up in Calcutta by Kartick Chandra Bose, a physician-entrepreneur, advertised its own products as being superior to imported stuff, because certain pills (such as lactic acid pills) deteriorated entirely by the time they were consumed in 'tropical' India.[71]

As far as the official medical opinion was concerned, when imports stopped, it was time to extend manufacturing within British India. The *IMG*, the official voice of the IMS, went to the extent of pointing out that inevitably Ayurvedic and other Indigenous medicine would integrate with 'scientific medicine': 'The need of the time is for us to set our own house in order and to range ourselves definitely on the side of science and truth if we do so, we can easily afford to live and let live; we have no desire to enter into a controversy with the worthy men who practice "systems" of medicine, for we know that all systems must in time die a natural death, or must merge in scientific medicine'.[72]

Therefore, the political momentum towards accommodating Indigenous systems of medicine within the infrastructure of the medical care offered by the state was contested robustly in official medical discourses. Nonetheless, once the medical services were provincialized after the reforms of 1919, the new Congress governments in the Upper Provinces and Madras attempted to legitimise Indigenous medicine by employing them at government-aided and local and municipal dispensaries.[73] Moreover, the princely states of

Gwalior, Bhopal, Cochin, Mysore, and Hyderabad patronised Indigenous medicine and appropriated both practitioners and their medicines into their official medical infrastructures.[74] In the devolved provincial legislatures, several governments debated and reflected on the usefulness of Indigenous medicines and the practicality of using Indigenous medical practitioners to fill the gaps in the medical services in the rural areas, which were too poor for a Western medical practitioner to consider. These did not always come to fruition, but in this brief period, the possibility seemed stronger than ever.

The GMS and the Cultivation of Substitute Medical Drugs: Digitalis

One example of the meandering policy of import substitution by the scientific cultivation of medicinal plants in India by the GMS is representative of this narrative from 1875 to 1944. One of the drugs that J.D. Hooker suggested in 1875 that could be grown easily in Indian hills was digitalis or foxglove, a European drug used in the treatment of heart disease. In the early 1920s, studies by R.N. Chopra and his associates at the Calcutta School of Tropical Medicine (henceforth CSTM) closely examined the potency and feasibility of the cultivation of digitalis and its manufacture in India. They found that *digitalis purpurea*, one of the four varieties in use in medicine, was first grown in ornamental borders in colonial hill stations. In the 1880s, the government botanical gardens at Saharanpur and Mussorie cultivated these for medicinal plants, but apparently, the produce was sparse, and it proved too expensive to harvest and process these. In 1913, the British-owned firm of Smith, Stanistreet and Co. of Calcutta, who were expanding their manufactured commodities at this time, made tinctures from digitalis from the government plantations to assess potency. The tests were inconclusive about the Nilgiri leaves. In the 1920s, the GMS sent samples to the CSTM where R.N. Chopra and his associates examined them and concluded that the Mungpoo (near Darjeeling) variety was deemed to possess active ingredients 'almost equal' to that of British and German varieties and that a variety grown 'for experimental purposes' in Kashmir was of similar, excellent quality. In 1928, the professor of chemistry at CSTM used the example of Indian digitalis to point out that locally grown drugs would need to be demonstrably potent as the active principles of drugs deteriorate in transit from Europe to India.[75]

In 1931, the DEC reported that digitalis was manufactured in India from local raw drugs and that the Kashmir state cultivated it systematically. However, medical men complained that its potency was variable, its active principles were notoriously unstable, and there was a great deal of variation in the methods of production. It was also pointed out that crude digitalis imported from abroad was often 'worthless and inactive, probably for having been robbed of their contents before import'.[76] In 1938, the newly established Central Research Laboratory examined 110 samples of digitalis marketed from several provinces in British India and found eighty-seven below the 80 per cent potency that was the international standard and fifty-seven samples with a potency lower than 50 per cent.[77] Although most of the samples were of Indian manufacture, the crude digitalis from which these were prepared would have been imported, in many cases, after having been denuded of its contents before shipment.

It was in 1940 when import shortages loomed once more that the government encouraged the formation of an Indian Chemical Manufacturers' Association, which was advised by R.N. Chopra. The Association's sub-committee on Indian drug cultivation pointed out yet again that 'if due attention is paid to the proper cultivation and utilization of vegetable drugs, India would not only be completely self-supporting in this respect but would also be able to develop an export trade'.[78] It identified digitalis (along with quinine and ephedrine) as foremost among the drugs that could be cultivated in large quantities in Indian conditions. In 1944, the IMS official in charge of Madras General Hospital pointed out that synthetic drugs were the future of medicine, but at the same time named digitalis as the example of the kind of drugs that India could usefully cultivate on a large scale after the war.[79]

The example of digitalis is representative of the attitude towards cultivating good-quality non-Indigenous drugs in India by the GMS. This veered between benign neglect and extreme urgency in times of shortage, interspersed with periods of activity occasioned by scientific research on the drug. Cinchona provides another example and follows a similar trend. The fate of the cultivation of cinchona in British India is better known because the government did establish plantations to cultivate the drug more systematically than any other.[80] One reason was that quinine was the one drug that the government tried to popularise through wide distribution both as prophylaxis and cure for endemic and epidemic malaria. The second and possibly more compelling reason for the government cinchona plantations was that, in the late nineteenth century India, when malaria epidemics were at their peak, an overwhelming proportion (c.97 per cent) of the cinchona grown globally was in the Dutch East Indies, with prices controlled by a small Dutch cartel.

The scarcity during the two world wars relit initiatives towards the cultivation of non-Indigenous (as well as Indigenous) drugs including digitalis and belladonna as their imports withered. Between the wars, despite a great deal of research at the CSTM and other institutions, there was not a great deal of acceleration in government or private cultivation of drugs scientifically. As we have seen in the previous chapter, the cause and possibilities offered by an Indian pharmacopeia, along with the concomitant use of Indigenous and locally produced drugs, continued to energise nationalists and medical professionals, some of them British. These lasted until the 1950s when the demand for botanical drugs was overshadowed by synthetic drugs and antibiotics.

Conclusion: The Forfeiture of the Promise of Import Substitution

The opportunities provided by the First World War did extend the scale and range of the manufactures of the GMS but in a very limited way. The GMS's largest venture was in the manufacture of quinine pills from the cinchona grown in the government plantations. The manufacturing units in Bombay and Madras offered little scope for new research on drugs or techniques of production. Nor did it use its advantages of scale and expertise to enhance the volume of production in medicines. Instead, once the war was over, it continued to depend on imports from British manufacturers, which were only supplemented by its own manufactures. Inevitably, it competed with local manufacturers, although GMS officials stoutly denied any competition.

More significantly, the GMS resisted pressure from within the government, as well as from Indian manufacturers and nationalist critics, because it rarely requisitioned finished products from local manufacturers. Local manufacturers, already facing stiff competition from renewed imports from UK and US after the war, found themselves out-manoeuvred by the GMS policies. In 1920, the British trade commissioner for India and Ceylon pointed out that after the war, Britain had regained its position and provided 50 per cent of the total drug exports to India, with the USA in second place.[81] It was also in this year that the government's Drugs Manufacture Committee, formed to enquire how Indigenous drugs can be used in manufacturing drugs within India, submitted its report. It pointed out that the Calcutta-based Smith Stanistreet and Company had greatly increased its range and volume of production during the war and was prepared to continue to manufacture drugs including digitalis, ipecacuanha, and strychnine from Indian sources if the GMS would stock their products instead of importing them. Meanwhile, firms that traded in raw drugs as well as manufactured products, such as Mysore Pharmaceuticals Ltd. (Mysore) and Messrs Sein Oberoi (Rawalpindi) sent a 'long list' of Indigenous drugs that they could supply to the GMS for the manufacture of therapeutic products.[82]

However, modest advances in enhancing the volume, quality, and patronage of Indian drugs and therapies were overwhelmed by the rush of imports of foreign drugs from industrialised nations including the UK, USA, Japan, and even Germany. Indian manufacturers united in protesting the absence of support from the GMS, which continued to buy most products from British firms, and the lack of tariff protection for Indian manufactures. The years after the war were especially fraught for the GOI, with nationalist rage at the massacre of Jallianwalla Bagh, price rises, and general disappointment at the meagre fruits of devolution of power.[83] One concession by the government to nationalist aspirations was the agreement to requisition as many products as possible from within India for government projects in all departments, including significant spending units like the railways and the Public Works Department. The government's Stores Department office was transferred from London to Delhi. This engendered some protection for Indian manufactures in iron and steel, small tools and machinery, and similar items.[84] But pharmaceutical and surgical products were very rarely requisitioned from within India by government departments on the grounds that the products manufactured locally were inferior in quality to imported ones. Government hospitals continued to requisition medicines centrally, through the director general's office and were unable to acquire anything from the local markets except temporarily during emergencies.

Private manufacturers complained bitterly about the GMS undercutting Indian manufacturers' rates for sale to hospitals and dispensaries and pointed out that the GMS benefitted from railway freight and alcohol tariff concessions. This enabled the GMS to unfairly price its commodities at just below the prices charged by private manufacturers.[85] The Indian Merchants' Chamber, with the indefatigable B.D. Amin, of Alembic Chemical Works Limited, sent a long memorandum to the Drugs Enquiry Committee in 1930.[86] Several manufacturing firms in Bombay and Calcutta similarly protested both the GMS's competition and its propensity to import therapeutic products instead of patronising local manufacturers. In response to the criticisms, in 1927, the Madras Store obtained the catalogues of 'two wholesale firms of chemists in India and one of the largest wholesale drug manufacturers in Great Britain' for the drug requirement of a large civil hospital in Madras.[87] It pointed out that the costs of supplying the civil hospital from the private suppliers were significantly more expensive than from the GMS, even conceding a 10 per cent increase in prices. The DEC pointed out that it was, in fact, the economies of scale –manufacturing for civil hospitals as well as the military institutions – that provided the key advantage in keeping costs down for the GMS. The DEC concluded that some complaints were partially justified, but in the interests of military security, advised that GMS continue to produce pharmaceutical preparations and import any therapeutic commodities if necessary. The GMS, therefore, continued to be the largest manufacturer and importer of drugs and pharmaceutical products in British India.

With the end of the shortage of imports after the First World War, the focus of legislation and official attention moved from controlling the 'superstitions' of Indigenous systems of medicine to the adulteration of drugs and therapeutic commodities. Public discourse and political challenges emphasised the lack of drug law in India, as they existed in Britain or the USA. The political battleground shifted the impurities in medicine to adulteration and wilful fraud. We will examine the movement for drug legislation in the next chapter.

5

Adulteration and the Medical Market

The push for an Indian pharmacopeia and greater use of locally available drugs were two aspects of the transformation of the drug market and its politicisation in nationalist discourse. Another was adulteration and its alternative, the purity, or authenticity, of drugs. Although there was a plenitude of therapies and treatments available, it was flooded with what the consumers, officials, and a large section of medical practitioners identified as adulterated medicine. The discourse of adulteration in colonial India encompassed not just drugs, but also several high-status commodities of consumption for sale: high-end, prized foodstuffs like milk and ghee, staples like rice, dal, mustard oil, wheat, or other grains, and the ready-made confectionaries and foods served at restaurants in colonial Indian cities.[1] With the discovery of vitamins between the wars, food and its constituents, and the nutrition derived from these, assumed significance in the public discourse.[2] From the mid-nineteenth century, the unwanted additions to common foodstuffs, or the corruption of foodstuffs and drinks were of concern to the elite British Indians. To the British and Indian elite, the 'bazaar', in this sense, represented everything that was dirty, contaminated, and, if transmitted to the relatively segregated British homes through contaminated substances, liable to produce disease.[3]

Among middle-class urban Indians to whom the adulteration of food, drink, and medicine remained an enduring apprehension, contamination was both a physiological and spiritual problem, threatening to disrupt the purity of the high-caste bodies that were sustained through structured rules of touch and rituals of ingestion. Food and drink have remained fundamental to political identities in modern India; scholars have reflected on the association of masculinity with meat-eating and, correspondingly, of the colonial discourse of effeminacy with rice-eating subjects.[4] The proliferation of restaurants and street food and the cheek-by-jowl existence and working lives with strangers of multiple castes and religions threatened the bodily purity and the sense of cosmic order among upper-caste Indians.[5] Yet, for most of them, living in crowded bachelors' boarding houses or in crammed *chawls* was essential to their livelihoods in the cities. Unable to control their environment outside the home and the body, the focus of their bodily regimens was instead fixed on adulterants from the outside-in – food, drink, and medicine that were handled by low-caste cooks and *halwais* in the restaurants and sweet shops; butchers, milkmen, oil-sellers, grocers, spice sellers, and the medicine sellers in the bazaars. With the rise of nationalism and the concurrent availability, as well as visibility, of packaged and branded medicine, the threat of adulteration or imitation/fake goods permeated to packaged commodities of both Indigenous and imported origins.

The high visibility of adulteration was reflected in the medical market as well. It led to contentious reflections on the reasons for these; all segments of the trade, from the small bazaar trader to the Indian manufacturing laboratories and British-Indian distributors and importers as well as medical practitioners of all hues, participated in emotive discussions on the nature of the trade and apportioned blame to the importers, Indigenous traders, or the Indian consumers who, it was said, were committed to cheapness over quality in the matter of drugs.

The Ambiguities of Adulteration

In the public sphere, 'adulteration' had several connotations, which sometimes overlapped. The category of adulteration, while quite clear to the consuming public as representing commodities that were not of the quality that they expected, in fact, hid several meanings and was used indiscriminately. Therefore, cases of poisoning, if not deliberate, were often defined as adulteration. Adulterants in food and drink were abundant. As scholars have pointed out, the use of adulterants identified low-caste vendors/suppliers and related to a complex framework of purity that encompassed the caste Hindu body and its functions. British medical men were similarly persuaded by the rhetoric of adulterants in foodstuffs; outbreaks of epidemic dropsy (often confused with what was later identified as beriberi) were, from the first outbreak in Calcutta in 1878, blamed on adulterants in mustard oil.[6] Other products commonly identified as adulterated were cosmetics and therapeutic goods where the packaging of a product was made to resemble the original, branded products and sold as such, and commonly found in the newly established brands for soap and toothpaste. Established brands in India often advertised and sent out flyers in English and regional languages to warn consumers and medical practitioners about 'imitation' medicine or toiletry.[7] Yet another category of adulteration was the sale of therapies in all forms that did not conform to the B.P. This was an ambivalent category and difficult to identify or prosecute. The B.P. was not the official pharmacopeia but it did serve as the unofficial mark of quality. The potency or the lack of adequate potency in any drug, therefore, was seen as adulteration in official, medical, and often public discourses. Since the potency of any therapy was often not labelled on the therapeutic products, there was distrust of any therapies available on the market. As far as Indigenous drugs were concerned, as we have seen, their potency and their active principles (or lack of these) were identified with the inefficacy of the drugs themselves. But where potency was an ambivalent category, every drug – Western or Indigenous – could be identified as adulterated.

This ambivalence was sustained by the legislative vacuum that encompassed both the content of therapeutic products for sale and the qualifications/training of the dispensers/medical practitioners themselves. Legislation to control both aspects evolved piecemeal and regionally. There was no food and drugs law in colonial India overall; laws regulating the sale of poisons and narcotics like cocaine evolved haphazardly. In Bengal, all pharmacists selling British pharmaceuticals containing any form of poison had to be registered, but this regulation hardly precluded hundreds of sellers from trading in the informal market. In Bombay, a similar act sought to restrict the sale of poisons but was largely ineffectual.[8] For medico-juridical purposes, provincial governments in Madras, Calcutta, and Bombay had appointed chemical examiners from the mid-nineteenth century whose duty, among many, was to examine food and other substances sold in the market and seized by the authorities, usually in cases of grave illness or the death of a consumer.[9] An all-India Poisons Act by the Government of India was only enacted in 1904 after a decade of deliberation; even here, its implementation was fragmentary at best.

Among the elite medical officials of the IMS, there were discussions on some regulation of the drug market. These began in the nineteenth century and continued until the inter-war years when British importers and Indian pharmaceutical companies successfully lobbied for a drug standardization committee, which presented its report in 1931. Its recommendations were not enforced until the Drug Act of 1944. Effectively, there was little or no control over the drug market in late colonial India. Adulteration, therefore, remained a catch-all term that encapsulated both the crude and processed drugs market until 1940.

In official discourse, the pre-existence of a large, informal market in variable drugs was supposed to have prevented any legislation to control it. At the first Indian Medical Congress at Calcutta in 1895, two IMS officials, including Chunilal Bose who served as chemical examiner to the Government of Bengal, read a paper together on the sale and 'ease of distribution' of poisons in India.[10] They pointed out that the chemical examiner in Calcutta and Madras had found hundreds of deaths by poisoning and urged for some kind of legal control. The Office of the Chemical Examiner was not new; the presidency of Bengal has established it in 1840 and other provinces followed by the middle of the nineteenth century. The duties of the chemical examiner extended to the examination and identification of cases of poisoning, both human and cattle; contamination in suspect foodstuffs and alcoholic spirits; and drugs, medicines, and cosmetics sold in the bazaars, and in other consumable products in the market.[11] At the turn of the century, British officials claimed that it was 'Utopian' for India to have a poison schedule similar to Britain's Drugs Act.[12] Even after the Indian Poisons Act was enacted in 1904, as the *Bombay Gazette* highlighted, only druggists selling B.P. products were covered under the terms of the law, whereas Indian medicines were exempt, and, moreover, 'Bunneahs and small dealers sell any number of drugs'.[13]

The Poisons Act (1904) referred only to poisons and specific narcotics and was mostly aimed at poisoning through arsenic, which was used in multiple ways in the everyday lives of ordinary Indians. The Poisons Act was, therefore, limited in scope and did not address the quality of drugs or other products that did not include specific, identifiable toxins. Any other drug, whether in an impure/adulterated state or imitations of original branded products, did not come under the legislation. These drugs varied in quality, their diversity a rich source of contention between competing British-Indian manufacturing firms as well as among Indian dealers. But the bulk of the blame for the preponderance of substandard products fell on the 'bazaar' traders, from the large wholesale importer to the modest pavement drug seller.

The market for adulterated (through fraud or accident) consumer products was vast and complex; complaints about adulteration in food, drink, cosmetics, and drugs abounded from the early nineteenth century. By the end of the century, with the established markets in urban India and the British manufacturing industry's aggressive advertising and sales in colonial markets, adulteration became the common trope for marketing British-manufactured therapies. In 1889, Charles W. White, the British agent for B.W. & Co., A.F. Pears & Co. and Burgoyne, Burbidges & Co. of England, claimed during a visit to England that German, French, and American competition, with full complicity of the Indian wholesalers, was marginalizing the British manufacturers with brazen adulterated oils and powders: 'calomel containing 50 per cent of chalk, santonin half boracic acid, sent here from France and Germany carriage paid and sold in the currency of the country, I fail to see how honest British competition can stand'[14] White successfully challenged the sale of an imitation of the popular Pears glycerine soap by dealers in Bombay as well as secured a fine of one thousand rupees to be paid by Messrs W.H. Nebel & Co. who was selling imitation Calvert's soap; both products allegedly supplied from Germany.[15] Next year, Bertie Smith, a British wholesale importer of drugs based in Bombay, identified 'German competition' as his problem and accused Continental firms of monopolising trade in certain drugs by exporting cheap, adulterated material to 'native' drug importers.[16] Similarly, the anonymous Indian correspondent of the *Chemist and Druggist* claimed that an 'American-made bazaar counterfeit' of an English-brand of patent drug made from sarsaparilla flourished in the Indian market.[17]

As we have seen in chapter 2, even British-owned importers dealt in diverse products, some of their own manufacture, and, due to their pre-established mercantile connections, supplied all major government departments. Naturally, these agencies acquired a reputation for purity and quality, not only

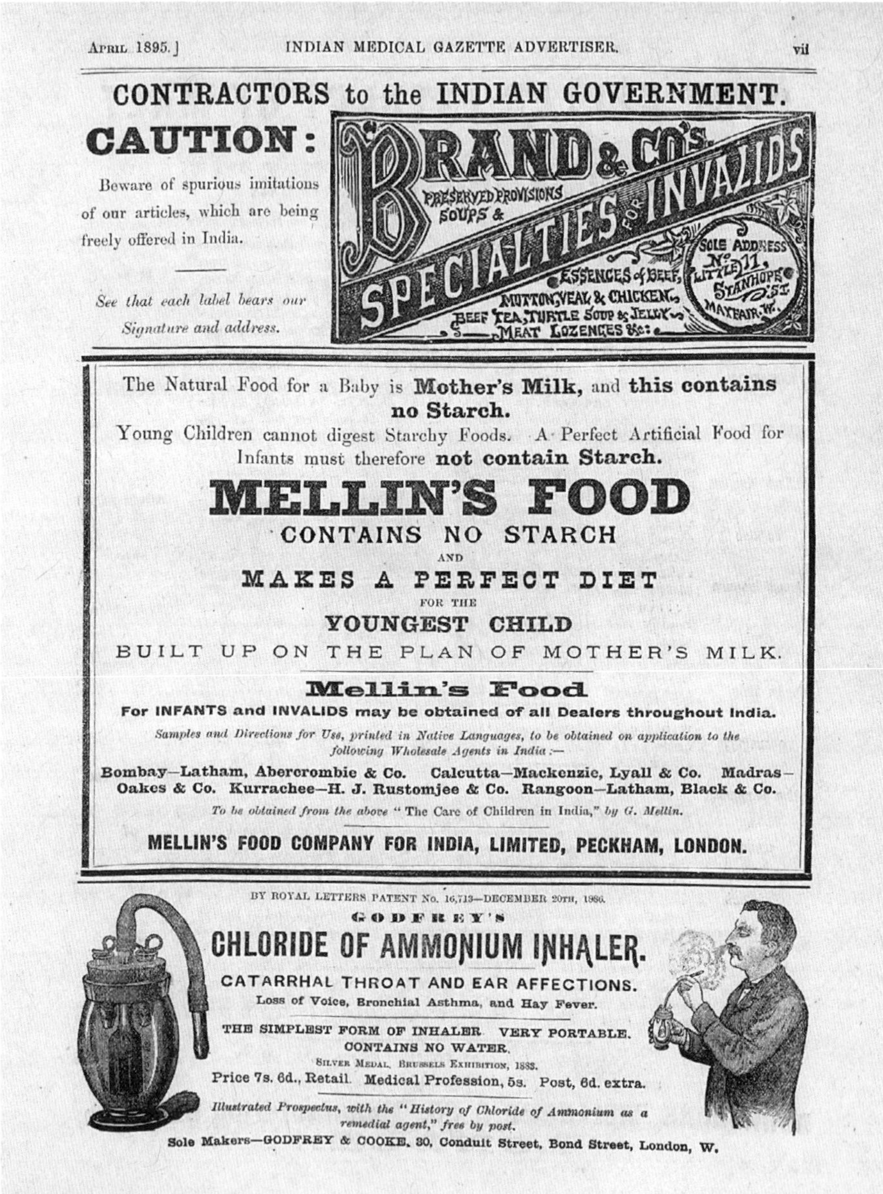

Figure 5.1 Advertisement for Mellin's food (*Indian Medical Gazette*, April 1895)

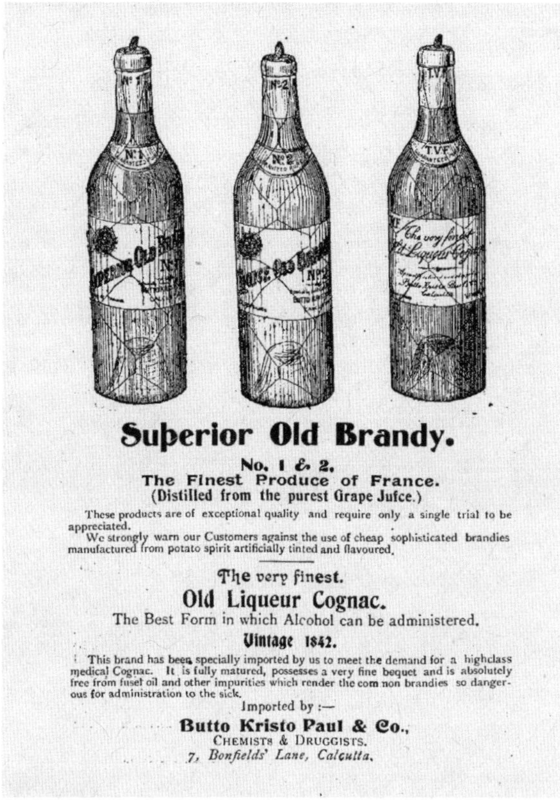

Figure 5.2 Advertisement for imported brandies, *Calcutta Medical Journal* 1, no. 3 (Sept. 1906)

among British residents but also among elite Indians who could afford to use their products. But even here, their products could arouse contention with the Indian drug importers carrying most of the blame for the inferior quality of patent medicines exported from Continental Europe.

Indian medical practitioners also participated in the discourse of adulteration. In 1905, the independent Parsi physician Dosabhai Rastamji Bardi, who taught at the Grant Medical College in Bombay, pointed out that adulteration prevailed on a large scale in several categories of food, cosmetics, and drugs in British India. His intervention identified exporters to India as the perpetrators of adulteration rather than retailers, whether British-Indian or 'bazaar'

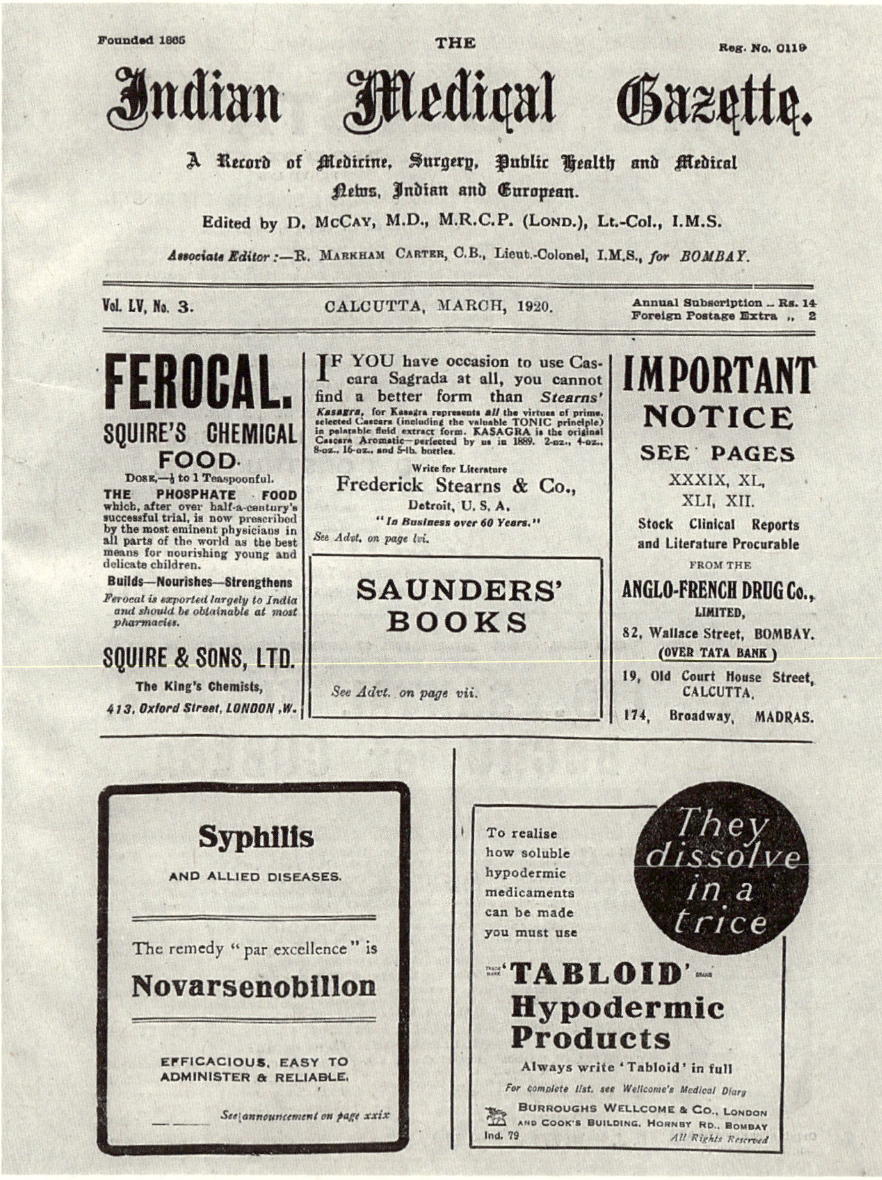

Founded 1865 THE Reg. No. 0119

Indian Medical Gazette.

A Record of Medicine, Surgery, Public Health and Medical News, Indian and European.

Edited by D. McCay, M.D., M.R.C.P. (Lond.), Lt.-Col., I.M.S.

Associate Editor:—R. Markham Carter, C.B., Lieut.-Colonel, I.M.S., *for BOMBAY.*

Vol. LV, No. 3. CALCUTTA, MARCH, 1920. Annual Subscription .. Rs. 14
Foreign Postage Extra „ 2

Figure 5.3 Miscellaneous medical advertisements in *Indian Medical Gazette*, March 1920

sellers. Citing records of the Chemical Examiners of Bombay from 1872 to 1902, Bardi claimed that there was consistent adulteration of commodities from Britain, the Continent, and America to the Indian market:

> It is necessary to remember that the retail druggist hardly adulterates them, but as people want cheap drugs, he buys adulterated articles … no wonder that medical men are disappointed in their treatment. Bombay, and for the matter … the whole of India, depends on European and American markets for their supply of drugs, at any rate of all important pharmaceutical and chemical preparations.[18]

Examples of adulteration in imports found by the offices of the Chemical Examiner and the Health Officer in Bombay included the presence of hydrochlorate of cinchonine, a much cheaper product, in a sample of quinine sulphate; potassium nitrate contained hydrochloric acid; worm tablets that did not contain any santonin; and a sample of tartar emetic that did not conform to B.P. tests.[19] Of more than a hundred examples of substandard imported products cited by Bardi, several had been provided not only to retail druggists but also to the Government Medical Stores by importers.

The sheer diversity and quantity of the therapeutic products on sale in India appeared to defy any serious attempt at regulation. As we have seen in previous chapters, a 'colonial addendum' to the B.P. of 1898 legitimised the substitution of several drugs for those that were easily available and commonly used in India by Western practitioners.[20] In chapter 3, we saw that this addendum was the consequence of a long campaign in India by several eminent medical personnel, both British and Indian.[21] British pharmacists alleged that the addendum was only of academic value:

> In India there is no Pharmacy Act; a Pharmacopeia is looked upon more as a guide … and the authoritative recognition of certain drugs, which, though used for centuries by the people of India, had never become commercial articles, was about as helpful as the omission of a number of drugs in daily use in every pharmacy in the East.[22]

Often the drugs sold in the market and labelled as B.P. standard were misleading because it was not illegal to market them and labelling was often wilfully misinformed. Therefore, manufacturers and distributors relied heavily on branding and advertising. All major drug manufacturers, both British and Indian-owned, warned against 'imitations' and substitutions cleverly produced to fool customers into buying substandard goods. What then defined purity to the customer? In a market where imported goods could be impure and substandard, the pricing of the goods provided guidance of sorts: expensive products were considered more efficacious. This standard was subverted regularly with the production of imitation drugs sold in reused packaging from reputable manufacturers.

Therefore, there was a wide spectrum between 'pure' and 'impure' drugs that embraced several degrees of authenticity. At this time, the public health movements that prevailed in India were focussed on sanitation and municipal improvement to minimise epidemics; the control of drugs (apart from poisons) was not a civil or government priority. The only drug that the government attempted to distribute widely in India was quinine and its alkaloids, at first for free, and then sold at a nominal price. Through inexpensive packets sold at post offices and, later, through a wide-ranging network of distributors including vaccinators and revenue collectors, various provincial governments sought to limit the devastation caused by malaria, especially during epidemics. As Patricia Barton has demonstrated, the high levels of adulteration (up to 80 per cent) of the quinine tablets sold by government agents and other distributors subverted the policy.[23]

Meanwhile, it was the Indian druggists who stocked the cheaper drugs and faced most of the blame for adulteration and substandard products in the market. These included imported patent medicines as well as drugs commonly used in both Indigenous and Western systems of medicine, such as belladonna, aconite, senna, and asafoetida. In 1910, the *British and Colonial Druggist* suggested that while, 'It would be unfair perhaps to say that quality does not count, but the native vendor is keen after a bargain … when it is said that he can purchase Easton's syrup in four oz. bottles, each packed in a carton at 36s. gross, it appears that the limit of cheapness has been reached'.[24]

Stung by the criticism in the Anglo-Indian and the regional press, the British-Indian importers and distributors pointed out that manufacturers in Britain and the Continent specifically produced low-quality commodities for the Indian market. Bathgate & Company, the oldest chemist and druggist retailer in Calcutta, clarified to the medical press that:

> We say that the majority of the British and Continental firms ship to Indian dealers very large quantities of drugs, the sale of which in England, Germany, France or the United States … would expose the vendors to prosecution, and which only remotely resemble the drug whose name they bear on, the labels as far as their physiological efficacy is concerned …
>
> India … is a cheap market … Every device to reduce the cost and secure business is practised – short weight, misdescription, imitation of labels and packing, and adulteration to a most astonishing extent. 'Anything is good enough for India' seems to be the motto of such shippers, and *Caveat emptor* their safeguard.[25]

The hugely popular Moore's medical manual remarked in its latest edition in 1916 that there was a great expansion of druggists' stores all over India and European expatriates could obtain many fresh drugs in the remote districts. Nevertheless, of the many locally available drugs at the village chemist's shop, it cautioned that 'the adulteration and sophistication of the specimens found in the Indian market, and the variability … of the drugs themselves owing to their being procured not from one but from many allied species, renders it quite impossible to use them with safety or economy'.[26]

Both from the 'legitimate' trade and from the official medical standpoint, the problem of adulteration was two-fold: the wilful dilution and imitation of standard drugs and proprietaries including the supply of cheaper varieties and the essentially large, uncontrollable, and uncertain quality of the fresh drugs on the market that problematized the Indigenous drugs market. A variant to this category was the deterioration of drugs in transit and due to climatic conditions, but these instances were subsumed in the broader category of wilful adulteration or dilution of drugs. Public discourse in India displayed a sporadic recognition that legislation was needed, and in the Upper Provinces, one Indian councillor even referred a request for legislation to the Select Committee in 1911.[27]

The discourse of adulteration was entangled with racial overtones and imperial dominance of the consumer market. Swadeshi manufacturers and the English and regional presses pointed out, in turn, that British, American, and Continental manufacturers produced substandard therapies specifically for the Indian market. As mentioned in chapter 3, *The Statesman* (Calcutta) began a campaign against spurious drugs in 1911 and alleged that diluted or impure drugs from Britain, the USA, Germany, and Japan were being imported on a large scale by distributors in India.[28] An intense debate ensued. Norman Hirst, a British pharmacist, alleged that 'they send out to India cheap varieties of quinine sulphates; compound extracts of sarsaparilla in some instances consisting chiefly of glucose and many other medicinal preparations ... are almost entirely deficient in active principle and are practically inert'.[29] He identified the complicity of both the consumers and exporters in this trade and especially indicated that the British-Indian companies that needed drugs on a large scale for their labouring populations, such as ' tea gardens, railway companies, collieries, ... send round "tender forms" or quotations for their medicines, and they usually accept the lowest tender'.[30] The problem of adulteration was, therefore, integral to the industry and the trade itself. The *Indian Medical Gazette*, which represented the medical fraternity of the IMS, agreed that there was widespread adulteration of drugs in India. Quinine, all vegetable oils including sandalwood and mustard, santonin, iodine, and alcohol-based tinctures were most affected. The *Indian Medical Gazette* pointed out that while the adulterated supplies were imported from England, North America, and Europe, 'These impure drugs are largely sold in India by small firms in the bazar and elsewhere'.[31]

With the increase in prices and scarcity during the First World War, adulterants in food and medicine became a visible problem in the cities. As with the poisons, legislation to curb adulteration was enacted piecemeal. In 1916, R. Braunfel, a commissioner of the Calcutta Corporation, introduced a bill for the prevention of food and drugs to be applicable to all municipal and districts in Bengal.[32] The bill was finally enacted in 1919 but referred only to adulterants in food and beverages. Similar political mobilisation within local governments and politics resulted in legislation on adulterants in food in Madras (1918), Bombay (1925), Punjab (1929), UP (1916), and in the Central Provinces (1919).[33] Srirupa Prasad has pointed out how the affective trope of adulteration engendered anxieties about the physical deterioration among the Bengali middle classes in late colonial India. She argues that in the lively Bengali public sphere 'alimentary anxieties' transcended the physical body and pervaded insecurity about the health and purity of several the Bengali nation, community, and selfhood.[34] As Saurabh Mishra has pointed out, anxieties about adulterants involved low-caste communities who sold the ritually pure commodities of milk and ghee, which were also used to make sweetmeats at the bazaars.[35] Brahminical ritual purity and the proliferation of prepared food in the bazaars coalesced and crashed in the cities of colonial India, eliciting complex discussions on adulteration, purity, and the self, both physical and metaphorical (of the 'community'/nation), health and prosperity, virility and masculinity.[36] These were undoubtedly informed by nineteenth-century colonial discourses of Bengalis as an emaciated, effeminate race.[37]

Significant as it was within nationalist imaginaries of the Bengali self, adulteration in consumable goods was not only a Bengali concern, even in Calcutta. Adulteration of food was a familiar issue within the influential Anglo-Indian (English) press and in the Hindi and Tamil presses as well; it was an all-India concern.[38] These concerns were linked to the new science of nutrition and the identification of a consumer market for vitamins and hormonal products such as insulin. Especially after the First World War, when micro-nutrients in food were discovered, synthesised, and marketed in the forms of tonics and pills, the distinction between commercial food/medicines/beverages grew ever blurrier. As local governments in urban India responded to the elite/upper caste's vocal protests about the poor quality of milk and ghee in the markets, a clutch of legislation at the provincial level was enacted. But these did not criminalise fraudulent marketing if it did not prove to be actively, physically harmful to the consumer. Even in that case, 'intent' had to be proved to ensure conviction. And the legislation still did not refer to drugs or therapeutic products, except poisons.[39]

The public sphere resonated with demands for control over poor-quality drugs and the deliberate introduction of adulterants in therapeutic products. Indian (as well as British) medical professionals were deeply involved in the discussions and medical journals as much as the lay press abounded in discussions on ways and means of ensuring the quality of therapeutic goods in the market. In the age of nationalist mobilisation, Western-trained Indian medical professionals often tended to view it at two levels: the failure of self-regulation by the merchants and industrialists, and the lack of professionalization by pharmacists. Both were instances of self-regulation and borrowed from similar solutions in Britain. The *IMR* argued for co-operative associations and suggested the organisation of 'co-operatives' as well as the establishment of an apprentice system to train prospective pharmacists.[40] It was not clear who were to organise the idyllic co-operatives – the traders, the Indian manufacturers, or the small minority of qualified pharmacists.

Adulteration and Disparate Dispensing

This lack of clarity was, in one respect, representative of the heterogeneity of medical practitioners and dispensers who prescribed and distributed medicines to their patients. There were no legal restrictions on who could practice medicine, after all. The Medical Registration Acts enacted in Bengal, Bombay, and Madras in 1912–14 were only intended to prevent unqualified doctors claiming Western medical training from being employed in government service or acting as medical witnesses in courts. Independent medical practitioners spanned across epistemic boundaries with the same ease with which they appropriated drugs and therapies from disparate sources. Most doctors dispensed medicines themselves as part of their practice, which included generic pills or tonics made in their workshops or dispensaries, or patented therapies advertised in every medical and lay periodical.

In 1864, Goodeve Chuckerbutty, one of the first Indians to train in Western medicine in Great Britain and secure in his self-worth as a legitimate medical graduate, had pointed out at the Bengal branch annual meeting of the BMJ that:

> Even the metropolis of India [Calcutta] is infested by a host of impudent harpies who prey upon the credulity of the unsuspecting. Every druggist and chemist, every apothecary and quack, every … fool, enjoys as yet full liberty to style himself a Doctor and prescribe for the sick … That any disappointed Sircar or worthless European may set himself up as a Medical practitioner by buying a few doses of quinine, castor oil, opium, and tartar emetic, and giving these out to the sick under false and bombastic names, is a grievous wrong to western medicine.[41]

Lately, historians have studied how the professionalization of medicine in India took place as medicine was 'vernacularized' or indigenised, especially in Bengal. Projit Mukharji has pointed out how 'daktari' or the profession of the 'doctor' as it emerged in late nineteenth-century colonial Bengal was constituted through the engagement of Western-trained Bengali doctors with Indigenous medical practitioners.[42] This 'nationalization' of Western medical systems occurred through emergent 'daktari' practices of borrowing from cultural idioms of the body and its care from Indigenous medical systems and assimilating these with knowledge of the human anatomy and cures delivered through modern therapeutic products and technology. For instance, Indigenous practitioners adopted the use of injections to deliver medicines in treatment or used the human pulse to measure heartbeat in diagnosis. Similarly, Western-trained practitioners advised yogic bodily regimes and Indigenous sick diets. Shinjini Das has shown that a plethora of medical practitioners of varying lineages and training prescribed homeopathic drugs that were novel and unique to Indian therapeutic cultures. In the process, homeopathy, a European system of medicine, was vernacularized by the public sphere, unique prescription cultures, and the local commercialization of its therapies by Indigenous family firms and in colonial Bengal.[43]

The process of vernacularization, useful though it is to understand Indigenous appropriations, implies a one-way relationship between Western drugs and Indian medical practitioners and consumers. It does not explain the significance that India held in the international search for Indigenous drugs to incorporate within Western pharmacopeia until the twentieth century. Similar appropriations of Western therapies and techniques/instruments of diagnosis were incorporated at other sites of non-European medical praxis, such as the traditional Chinese medicine (TCM) or local Sino-Vietnamese medicine.[44] Nor does vernacularization adequately explain how the international drugs trade infiltrated and hybridised medical therapies and practice on a global scale in this period.

As indicated elsewhere in this book, it is essential to complicate the divides between the Indigenous and the Western therapeutics on which the arguments for vernacularization reside. This, in turn, helps us to understand why the problem of adulteration existed across the therapeutic spectrum of the Indian market. To start with, until the 1920s, there was not a great deal to distinguish Western therapies from Indigenous ones. As seen in chapter 3, drugs from the Indian bazaar were continuously adapted to Western pharmacopeia and substitutions or replacements were carefully presented. As the *Indian Medical Gazette* editorialized in 1879 there was a:

> Practical and useful threefold classification of the medicinal products of India, namely (1) pharmacopceial drugs indigenous to or procurable in India; (2) non-phar- macopoeial drugs used in Native medicine, and (3) medicinal substances whose properties have not been as yet investigated nor their applications in disease defined.[45]

Although the quest for an Indian pharmacopeia was not fulfilled in colonial India, the inclusion of Indian drugs into Western pharmacopeia occurred parallel to the indigenization of Western drugs, particularly through methods of delivery (pills, injections, bottles) and marketing strategies (advertisements in print media in multiple forms and languages). In crude form, there were hundreds of common drugs in between Western pharmacopeia and bazaar drugs.

In colonial India, the public sphere was crowded with medical practitioners' interventions in public debates, offering varying degrees of medical authority and knowledge. Debates on masculinity or effeminacy; the necessity or otherwise for bodily purity and continence among (male) nationalists; the suitable age for marriage, sexual intercourse, and reproduction for girls or women were all up for debate, involving medical experts of all persuasions as well as political workers, educationists, and social reformers. Western medical practitioners and many prominent vaids and hakims participated in these debates and found relevance in the public sphere on account of their ability to process Indian cultural norms of the body to Western medical practises and, in turn, translate Western therapeutic praxis into forms that were meaningful in the social and cultural worlds of (largely upper-caste) Indians. Historians have focussed on the medico-cultural debates and conflictual moralities that colonial modernity generated among literate Indians. The acceptance of Western medicine, however, occurred not just at the site of the public iterations of the ideal national Indian bodies of men and women. The extent of consumption of these commodities depended on the range, quality, and quantities of the commodities in the market. The most visible element in this market was the therapies on sale.

Therefore, the indigenization or vernacularization and 'nationalization' of medicines in colonial India were the reflection of the unregulated market where such experiments in 'braiding' and mixing medical technologies and drugs were possible.[46] This heterogeneity characterised medicines as well as much of the medical professions, including doctors, hakims, and homeopaths as well as apothecaries, dispensers, and itinerant pill pedlars in India. Professionalization, as understood in the Western experience, did not occur until after the government legislated drug control laws after 1940, and only in a fragmented way thereafter. There was a thin line between heterogeneity and adulteration of drugs in the market. The sale of adulterated, cheap medicines flourished in the absence of drug control legislation and because the private drugs market catered to those with fewer means as well as the more affluent.

Legislating Adulteration

The problem of adulteration reinvented itself with the new urgency for drug control in the twentieth century. The popular movement for a drug control policy continued in the Indian press, both national and regional. In 1925, an article in the daily *The Bengalee*, an English language moderate nationalist daily, alleged that all reputed pharmaceutical companies in Calcutta, both British-owned and Indian, made a regular practice of misleading customers by labelling their products as being of B.P. strength, including BCPW, Stanistreet, Smith & Co., D. Waldie & Co., and B.K. Paul. It claimed that the Chemical Examiner of Calcutta had reported that 'local firms in competition with one another and with the importing firms try to reduce the manufacturing cost by using less medicament and alcohol, and that the importing firms in their turn have begun a similar practice'.[47] The piece caused mayhem. It was reprinted in the *Statesman*, which, as we have seen, had initiated a campaign against drug adulteration in 1911. After a strong protest from Stanistreet, Smith & Co., the *Indian Medical Record* retracted the piece. But the all-pervasive collusion of manufacturers, producers, and distributors in various stages of adulterating drugs was apparent and raised continual pleas for a food and drugs act for India in the medical and the general press.

During the First World War, several Indian manufacturers particularly the large producer-retailers, made a fortune in supplying government contracts. The Indian army itself was deployed at several places in Mesopotamia, imports from Europe proved difficult, and those from Germany ceased altogether. The GMS's produce proved inadequate; it relied on manufacturers based in India to provide several standard drugs and surgical products. British-Indian importers/manufacturers including Smith Stanistreet & Co. (Calcutta), D. Kemp & Co. (Bombay), as well as newer companies such as Bengal Immunity (Calcutta) benefitted from the virtual cessation of imports.[48] Immediately after the First World War, the Smith Stanistreet & Co. moved to new, larger premises that accommodated both their factory and large retail outlet. Yet, even here, the problems of variations in the potency of medicine and the quality of surgical products persisted. In 1916, the RAMC blacklisted the Bombay-based British-Indian manufacturer Phillips & Co. for providing the British Army in Mesopotamia with surgical dressings that had little or no antiseptic content and, therefore, violated its terms of contract.[49] As we have seen in chapters 3 and 4, the promise of 'import substitution' and a deeper exploration of indigenous drug plants (shorn of their 'impurities') by medical men and entrepreneurs alike enabled the complexity of the market to intensify rather than become simplified and streamlined, as Western medical professionals had hoped. The huge range of Indigenous drugs and the local manufacture of drugs came to official and medical notice more vividly, and the public discourse and medical disquiet on the lack of regulation in the market grew in the inter-war period. At this time, the UK and Europe-based companies were accused of dumping their outdated surplus articles on the Indian market.

The Government of India set up a biochemical standardisation laboratory in 1937 in Calcutta. In 1939, the laboratory found that of 130 samples of liquid ergot, used in emergency haemorrhage cases, 112 were substantially below strength, and fifty-eight had no active principles evident in them. Both locally manufactured and imported drugs were implicated. Of the samples examined, 103 were local, and twenty-seven were of foreign manufacture. The *IMG* pointed out that 'that an inferior quality of both crude and finished preparations of ergot, unsaleable in their countries of origin due to stringent drug laws, is being purchased in India at a cheap price'.[50]

Feeding the confusion over adulteration was the heterogeneity of the market itself. This heterogeneity was manifest in the therapeutic commodities as much as in the knowledge, experience, and qualifications of medical practitioners and dispensers themselves. The spectrum of medical products in the Indian market reflected the range of medical practitioners and their changing crafts as well as the literate, self-medicating consumers. The principal manufacturing firms in Calcutta, Bombay, and other metropolises offered a range of products that used formularies from both 'Western' and 'Indigenous' traditions. The vibrant print cultures and the emergence of the literate and self-aware middle-class Indian, therefore, joined and informed the content of medical writings in the medical and general presses.

The incremental number of Indian and imported self-help prescription manuals and more formal academic works on materia medica that also flooded the market in this period was underscored by the intense trade in pharmaceutical products. These publications were inundated with advertisements for a bewildering array of therapeutic commodities and instruments – from pills and powders to syrups and tonics, instruments for extracting 'meat juices', dried milk and eggs, vitamins, and hormonal products. The possibilities for 'adulterants' in the foodstuffs as well as medicines were seemingly infinite.

There were distinct trajectories of adulteration in the drug market. Indian manufacturers presented their therapeutic products as both physically and culturally more suitable vis-à-vis imports. Indian manufacturers were reinforced by claims from vaids, hakims, and even a few Indian doctors that imported drugs were materially and culturally unsuitable for use in India. The claims were based on two fronts; first, that several products from the UK or North America deteriorated in quality and declined in potency during the maritime passage to India, whereas local products were fresher and provided the potency that their labels indicated. This was an established criticism. Indeed, the degradation in the quality of the medicines brought from the UK had initially occasioned the use of local and bazaar medicines by the surgeons of the first Navy hospitals in British India. Although the shipments arrived faster now, the long-held views about the heat and moisture of the tropics and their adverse effect on medicines persisted in medical discourse. Indigenous suppliers could claim that their goods were more reliable and superior. Related to this was the older, Orientalist discourse of the characteristic, distinct tropical body. This discourse had a rich and tenacious life; from the eighteenth-century European medical thought reflected on the tropical climate and correspondingly to the legitimacy of local medicines for tropical (native) constitutions.[51] The arguments shifted emphasis and acquired overlapping implications. Racial distinctions remained significant, but arguments for 'seasoning' or adaptability of white bodies in the tropics declined. Local or Indigenous medicines were loaded with not just cultural heft and historical meaning, its enthusiasts pointed out the advantages of fresh and, therefore, more 'active' effects. As late as 1938, an Indian pharmacologist trained in London pointed out that in certain circumstances, local Ayurvedic drugs were more convenient and efficacious as Western preparations of the same drug.[52] Therefore, decayed/deteriorated medicines and adulteration led to a campaign for Indian medicines.[53] Even the Secretary of State's office in London, heavily biased in favour of British exports in the late nineteenth century, advised the Government of India against the purchase of elastic syringes for children as they 'deteriorate in the hot climate'.[54]

The second claim of adulteration was directed towards proprietary drugs and their contents. This referred to proprietary medicines that were imported, mostly from the UK and North America, and available at the reputed, established end of the medical market. Proprietary medicines were also locally manufactured across the spectrum of Western and Indigenous medical therapies. The so-called patent and proprietary medicines formed a substantial part of the drug market in colonial India. There was no patent law in India until 1911; even then, the so-called patent medicines were not formally patented as such.[55] They referred to all preparations with secret content, i.e., they were packaged materials whose constituents were not public. Patent and proprietary remedies were widely used. In a medical market where self-help manuals for diagnosis and treatment were common, advertisements in print media plentiful, and multiple layers of medical practitioners and dispensers were rife, packaged proprietary medicine for specific ailments could create a huge demand.[56] This demand originated both from the practitioners and dispensers as well as from the consumers.

Proprietary remedies and their overstated, often ludicrous, claims were common in Great Britain and indeed, in the USA in the nineteenth century. As the medical occupations formalised their distinct skills and services, pharmacists formed their own self-regulatory bodies, and doctors and pharmacists campaigned extensively for drug control legislation and surveillance over the claims of medical advertisements and proprietary medicines. In the early twentieth century, the British Medical Association and the Royal College of Physicians debated the ethical boundaries of the claims made by manufacturers of proprietary medicines and went to the extent of publishing the (widely used) ingredients of the most popular proprietary remedies sold on the market and gave evidence to the Select Committee on the Sale of Patent and Proprietary Medicines in 1912.[57] Historians have pointed out that qualified physicians' monopolization of the practice of medicine and their delegitimizing of medicines manufactured by chemists as quackery were due to the rivalry and conflict over consumer-patients.[58] Of course, the line between the hypothetical ethical physician and the commercially minded drug seller was not entirely clear cut, especially in the poorer regions, for instance, physicians dispensed medicines and doubled as shopkeepers in Scotland in the early twentieth century.[59] The narratives of professionalization of medical experts in Britain would not be replicated in British India. As we have seen in the previous chapters, medical cultures and the relationship between consumers and the medical market in India represented a strand of colonial modernity, and its contours would not fit into the palimpsest of the praxis of medicine and the market in the metropolis. Nonetheless, the need for a set of rules to regulate the quality of the medical commodities that swamped the market in colonial India became urgent and clear during and after the First World War. When the Government of India experienced international pressure to restrain the trade in narcotic drugs (at the time sold in pharmacies), it instituted the Drugs Enquiry Committee (DEC) in 1930.

The Long Half-life of the DEC Report

In the inter-war period when the Health Committee of the League of Nations initiated international cooperation on both the control of narcotic drugs and the standardization of sera and vaccines, the Government of India gave in to the general clamour at home as well as to the new international initiatives. It formulated and passed the Dangerous Drugs Act (1930) that enforced control over trade in drugs derived from Indian hemp, coca leaves, and opium.[60] More significantly, it also instituted the DEC. The committee was chaired by R.N. Chopra, who had extensively researched the properties of Indigenous drugs at the Calcutta School of Tropical Medicine. The committee was to devise a system of legislating all drugs, Indigenous and Western, as well as recommend ways to institutionalise the drug-dispensing professions in all of British India. The DEC submitted its report in 1931. The report was comprehensive and its recommendations were clear and simple. It arrived at these through consultation with the nascent industry, retailers, government medical officials, pharmacists, and independent medical practitioners. The report made recommendations to regulate the import, sale, and manufacture of pharmaceutical products in the country and to streamline the training of pharmacists in technical institutes.

In this final section, we will see how the committee's report attempted to consolidate and make uniform the impossibly plural drug industry. It provided, for the first time, an informed overview of drug production and dispensing in government and private hands throughout India. The DEC report had a long shelf life; the central government acted on the bulk of these recommendations only when it passed the Drug Act in 1944. At first glance, the delay in implementing the recommendations of the DEC for more than a decade seems normal; after all, most reports of the Government of India were commissioned to elicit information and they rarely inspired clear-cut action by the government. The Indian Industrial (Holland) Commission report (1918) was case in point. It was convened during the First World War to examine the conditions for industrialisation in British India. The recommendations of the Committee, including legislation for industrial safety and labour laws and the establishment of an India-wide chemical service, were mostly ignored once the war was over.[61] The newly constituted provincial governments did set up a separate department of industries and made a few gestures to promote technical education but these instances were rare and limited to specific industries and skills, such a railway 'workshop' technical school in Lucknow.[62]

The DEC was established partly in response to Western nations' aims to curtail trade in narcotic goods (cocaine and opium) between the wars through the agency of the League of Nations. The prospect of the standardisation of drugs within British India was a relatively minor digression from controlling the free flow of opium or cocaine products for recreational use and manufactured by pharmaceutical firms in Europe.[63] By the 1930s, the Geneva Convention on narcotics had settled on policing the trade/export and supply of narcotic drugs. One reason for the halting progress on the recommendations of the DEC was that the colonial government was politically invested in the narcotics trade. Once the diplomatic arrangements for policing international trade in narcotics were established, it was reluctant to place any further checks on the drugs trade, especially given the large proportion of British exports of drugs and chemicals to India.

Controlling the drug market was a complicated affair. As we have seen, the unregulated elements included multiple drugs from differing epistemic frameworks, a large and variegated set of producers and manufacturers, as well as several categories of medical practitioners and drug dispensers. Moreover, by no means were these categories mutually exclusive. Above all, drug control was expensive; apart from establishing central and provincial drug testing/standardisation laboratories, some government medical colleges would need to offer diplomas in pharmacy to train dispensers. Legislative action would be required at the central and provincial levels to regulate the medical professions. Any determined effort to regulate the trade would require a clear judgement of how to assess Indigenous drugs and those that did not belong to the BP. The government would also finally have to legislate Indigenous therapies, their training methods, and their diplomas rather than rely on their corporate bodies to regulate these. Most of these would require financial resources and political will. With the government's declining finances after the crash of 1929, and the strong nationalist alliances of the Ayurvedic and Unani organisations at this time, this promised to prove difficult and contentious.

Once the report was published, the Government of India consulted with the provinces on the specific points of standardisation of laboratories, inspection of factories, establishment of medical colleges to train pharmacists, and the advisability of controlling Indigenous drug production. Most provincial governments cavilled at the cost, some flatly declaring that these could not be funded provincially. Smaller provinces, like Coorg, declared that it could 'ill-afford' a pharmacy council and did not have a single medical college.[64] The Assam government pointed out that the formation of an Indian pharmacopeia or a pharmacy council, or assessing the clinical value of Indigenous drugs, were best done by the federal government.[65] Several provinces voiced dismay at the prospect of losing excise revenue income if, following the recommendations of the DEC, they stopped imposing excise duties on alcohol-based medicines.

Even more significantly, the Royal Society of Medicine in London objected to implementing most of the recommendations of the Report, including an Indian pharmacopeia; 'The proposal to create an IP is one which cannot be too strongly deprecated. The world needs fewer, rather than more pharmacopeia, and to add another national pharmacopeia to the existing number, would be a retrograde step'.[66] It also objected to the inspection system for drug manufacturers in India, arguing that India did not yet have enough trained chemists to usefully benefit from these. The Society was not keen for British drug manufacturers to lose their Indian markets as credible drugs legislation would guarantee the quality of the relatively cheaper and easily available Indian therapeutic products and challenge the near-iconic status of British medical commodities.

The central government did formalize a drug standardisation centre in Calcutta, headed by R.N. Chopra. The Benares Hindu University offered degrees in pharmacy from 1937, admitting twenty students annually.[67] The rough and ready 'compounders' – unqualified dispensers – who acted as pharmacists in most dispensing stores numbered around 27,000 at this time. They carried the burden of the ill fame of the dispensing profession, as did the Indigenous *dais* (midwives) who were caught between halfhearted attempts to regulate their profession by the government and qualified medical practitioners.[68]

Attempts on the part of the government to begin regulating the drug trade included the introduction of a Drugs Import Bill in 1937. It was intended to control the import of foreign drugs, especially those 'misbranded' and, as the federal government explained, was not intended to 'interfere in the legitimate drugs trade'.[69] The Indian Merchants' Chamber, the most influential association of Indian entrepreneurs with strong nationalist ties, cautiously welcomed the proposed legislation but pointed out that to be effective, the legislation needed to be extended to princely states and encouraged the provincial governments to enact similar legislation for Indian manufactures:

> As however, the bill extended only to British India … necessary that imports of drugs and medicines to Indian States should be similarly controlled, and that to this end, efforts to secure passing of similar legislation by Indian States in their jurisdiction should be made. They also suggested the necessity for having provincial legislation for controlling similarly manufacture and sale of drugs and medicines within the country.[70]

It was resisted by Indian manufacturers and traders, who insisted that this act would delegitimise *all* Indian manufactures; 'The Drug Bill now in the Assembly is defective … and if passed into law would put Indigenous products under a stamp of inferiority and thereby prejudice the growth of the indigenous industry'.[71] The bill was subsequently dropped. It was not until the

Second World War disrupted the import of all commodities including essential drugs into India and exposed how dependence on imports endangered civil servants and the urban elite, that the government tabled the Drugs Bill of 1940 and finally accepted most of the recommendations of the DEC. These were legislated formally in 1944, setting the standards for manufactured drugs and the control of medical practitioners and pharmacists.

6

Disparate Dispensing
Pharmacy in the Eclectic Market

The medical market was formed through traders, manufacturers, government officials, medical experts, and a medley of public-leaning writers and speakers. Of these, one category of individuals who were deeply invested in the drug trade and yet were little noticed in the public sphere was the dispensers of medicine. Yet the preparation and sale of every therapeutic commodity rested on their skills and experience, and the moments between handing a written prescription (or more often, proffering a verbal query) and handing over a package of pills, powder, bottle, or ointment were crucial to the medical expert and the consumer alike. In the one hundred years from the mid-nineteenth century to Indian Independence, the establishment of hospitals and the expansion of the medical market transformed the roles of dispensers in the dispensaries and vaids' or hakims' consulting rooms. This transformation of the roles of the dispenser was not unique to India. In Great Britain, the transformation from the trade of the apothecary to the profession of the pharmacist is framed through the narrative of professionalisation and medical specialism.[1] This narrative fits well enough into a reading of a self-regulating body in civil society, consisting of qualified individuals who settled into their respective positions within a shifting hierarchy of specialisms in the nineteenth century.

Such narratives are unavailable in colonial contexts. Just as the profusion of Indigenous drugs defied standardisation, for pharmaceutical dispensers of differing skills, knowledge, and legitimacy, the journey towards professionalisation remained incomplete or inadequate. This was as true of purveyors and dispensers of 'scientific' medicine as of the numerous other retailers of therapeutic products. The dispensers ranged from those with a qualification legitimised by the Royal College of Pharmacists and employed in army hospitals to the much-derided itinerant pedlars who mainly traded in generic powders that were made of a mixture of, for example, asafoetida, dried ginger, and a little opium and sold cheaply as a panacea for all ills. There has been a trajectory of professionalisation of pharmacy in modern India; however, it has been uneven and desultory. Instead, a profession with a hybrid nomenclature and requiring eclectic skills has flourished – that of a compounder. A *compounder* was a term initially employed for dressers in military hospitals. Later, the role expanded to include helpers who prepared and mixed the medicines at the chemist and druggists' stores, sometimes at the direction of a qualified pharmacist.

There is little attention to the position or the role of the compounder in the medical history of India. Subaltern perspectives on medicine and the state have focussed on Indian inoculators or sanitation workers as agents in the new public health regimes of the colonial state.[2] Or historians have reflected on how public health regimes instigated nationalists to mobilise politically against the state's coercive policies of restraint or quarantine during the plague.[3] The sanitation worker has been understood as a subaltern resister when striking over the non-payment of their modest wages or the abysmal features of their work.[4] Scholars have, instead, explored the Indigenous or the subaltern experience of translating, encountering, and/or appropriating Western medicine to the person of doctor/daktar/vaid/baidya/hakim or homeopathic 'doctor'. Mukharji, for instance, has explored the experience of the appropriation of small technologies within modern Ayurvedic praxis. He terms this as a version of the 'techno-modernity', which is also used by Joseph Alter to discuss the postcolonial globalisation of yoga. And indeed, as Mukharji points out, in the case of practised Ayurveda, the status implied in the words 'tradition' or 'modern', or indeed the 'global' and the 'local', is inaccurate and the binaries they represent are not analytically useful.[5]

To understand the translation or praxis of medicine in colonial India, Mukharji has presented vernacularisation as a version of provincialisation of Western medicine, and demonstrated how a pocket watch, microscope, or stethoscope could be incorporated into a multi-layered epistemic framework of Ayurvedic medical practice in colonial Bengal, thereby accommodating differing notions of the human body and its temporal rhythms. He also argues that the 'daktars' or Indigenous (Bengali) medical practitioners generated a form of pluralistic 'daktari' medicine as physicians in the lower echelons of the official hierarchy within the dispensary system in nineteenth-century north India.[6]

Scholars have posited vernacular science as an alternative to Western science; as transgressive and challenging hegemonic scientific expertise.[7] Or they have argued for vernacular knowledge (assumed as orally transmitted) as a postcolonial alternative to mainstream scientific knowledge. In the latter case, Helen Tilley has defined vernacular knowledge as situated in language and culture (and place, presumably), and has suggested that it represents 'the translation and, more important, appropriation of select dimensions of vernacular knowledge into scientific worldviews'.[8] The assertion that Indigenous systems of medicine (for instance, Ayurvedic/Hakimi practice) were not static and had a dynamic relationship with what was understood as scientific medicine in nineteenth-century India offers a corrective to Tilley's somewhat unilateral approach to vernacularity.

However, in these various discussions of praxis and ingenious skills, the ubiquitous compounder in every chemist/retail unit or dispensary has not received much scholarly attention. Despite its politics of selective appropriation, by its very definition, the vernacular stands for a mime, in this case, a lesser version of the standard and the normative medical science in the extant historiography of colonial India. In the work of both Das and Mukharji, vernacular medicine refers to and emphasises the Indigenous, and the theme of vernacularisation of Western medicine has so far suggested selective epistemic and *cultural* appropriations of Western medical discourses and practices. In Mukharji and Das' schemes, the vernacular as a social category has been used as a relatively elite one, denoting physicians or the medical literati. In the nineteenth century, the traditional high-status Unani practitioners in north India, for instance, rued the self-trained *neem hakim* ('semi-doctors') who appeared pervasive in Urdu popular print.[9] Yet these adaptations were embedded in language and print and their visible aesthetics were available on packaging or in presentations. Perhaps because the compounders occupied the interstitial and, thereby, indistinct ground between the physician and the sanitary workers, they have often been written out of the history of Indian medicine. Vernacularisation and reconstitution of medicine occurred at multiple social sites, not always involving the translation of Western therapies.

The eclecticism in the Indian medical market extended to medicines themselves and the methods of extraction and blending of these (like diagnostic practices) with extant therapies. While respectable Indigenous practitioners acknowledged these influences, there were others whose borrowings were stealthier and more pervasive. There was no formal requirement for any qualification to be employed as a pharmacist, and indeed there was no separate diploma or degree in pharmacy available in the Indian medical colleges until the mid-1930s. Even in the larger European pharmacies, there was usually just one British pharmacist with a degree from Britain to show for his enhanced status and wages. The mixing or preparations of the drugs themselves was undertaken by a slew of Indian subordinates, most of whom were classed as *coolies*, a generic term for a manual labourer. This term, as well as that of the compounder, encompassed a range of roles and variations in knowledge of drugs and an array of acquired technical skills. The new occupation of compounder emerged with the expansion of retail dispensing from medical stores and the extension of the 'independent' or private medical practice.

The Compounder and the 'Independent Medical Practitioner'

As far as the medical consumer at the bazaar was concerned, there was little distinction to be made between the dispenser and the doctor; both provided medical advice and medicines for a price. The 'independent medical practitioner' was how the military and official medical men described the graduates from the new medical colleges in the presidency capitals.[10] These Indian graduates with diplomas in Western medicine comprised the largest proportion of doctors practising Western medicine in British India. Some among them were employed in government service at a rank termed 'hospital assistant' or sub-assistant surgeon' in the government hospitals or aided hospitals when these expanded in the mofussils in the late nineteenth century. These men, employed in what was known as the 'subordinate medical services' in government, provided the bulk of the everyday medical services for hospitals and dispensaries, with IMS surgeons and assistant surgeons performing supervisory roles. The IMS remained, by and large, the preserve of the British until the Great War, and even then, the entry of Indians (thinly disguised as blocking graduates of substandard Indian medical colleges) was contested deeply by British medical and military officials.[11] The government medical officials were also allowed to practise privately for fee-paying patients outside their consulting hours in the hospitals or dispensaries, and this put them, and especially the subordinate services' officials, in direct competition with the so-called independent doctors who earned their living entirely in private practice. The compounder, originally an occupation of an assistant to the apothecary in the Indian army, added another layer to this spectrum of practitioners of Western medicine. Their exact role is difficult to identify because most of them performed several roles and had formal skills in few or no areas – dispenser, dresser, medical adviser at the dispensary, medical practitioner, or 'doctor' – their roles were informal and indispensable.

Most medical colleges in India produced qualified practitioners of Western medicine who depended on private practice and lived in the expanding cities and towns in British India. It was predominantly the Indian doctor who had obtained a qualification termed 'Vernacular Licentiate in Medicine and Surgery' who involved himself in translating and popularizing elements of Western medicine through private practice. As Mark Harrison pointed out, until the provincial Medical Registration Acts (1912–14), the profession was more or less unregulated, and even the acts only barred medical professionals from Indigenous systems and unlicensed medical colleges from government service or court appearance as medical experts and from issuing sick notes for government employees.[12] Therefore, in the late nineteenth century, the private 'licenciate' of the medical colleges found himself in direct competition with men of differing experiences and knowledge, all of whom styled themselves as Western-style 'doctors'. These included retired military apothecaries/pharmacists and young men from the newly established private medical colleges who may have passed some, but not all, of their medical examinations to qualify for their diplomas. They often included entirely unqualified men who may have familiarised themselves with mixing Western medical powders or preparing tinctures and unguents by working as compounders at retail chemist and druggists' stores. Since there was no law against practising medicine, the professional lines between the druggist/pharmacist/compounder and the doctor and even the vaid/hakim were blurred. Of course, even in Britain, where the Medical Registration Act of 1858 had mostly settled professional boundaries, general physicians in poorer areas often supplemented their modest incomes by mixing and dispensing medicines from their own medical stores.[13]

The skills of the compounder/assistant pharmacists who served as chemists/ druggists in Indian retail medical stores were those of specialists who stocked, mixed, extracted, pounded, diluted, and added solvents and, occasionally, adulterants. The pharmacist's occupation and status in colonial India were highly stratified at the same time as being fluid, with the inclusion of Fellows of the Royal Pharmaceutical Society who worked for the great British-Indian manufacturers/distributors in the metropolises to the keen-eyed *pansaris* (drug collectors and sellers) in the bazaar. Even in the established European pharmacies, the official pharmacist had only a supervisory role:

> In Bengal and the Punjab … the European … copies the prescription in the book, and at the same time calls out the ingredients to a native, who is called a 'compounder'. He has served a sort of an apprenticeship in some dispensary, then has some experience in a drug store, and there develops into a compounder. He seldom speaks English, but, as a rule, can make out the names of the ingredients and quantities, but can seldom read directions. He places all his bottles on the counter, and then prepares the prescription while the European gives him the quantities. Unless the prescription requires some special preparation, he manages to compound it all right; They do everything – prepare plasters, suppositories, etc., make all the preparations for the shelves-but everything must be checked. After the prescription is compounded, he calls out the quantities, and has his bottles in order as they appear in the prescription.[14]

The qualified and trained pharmacist in the European stores was a figurehead and the dispensing of prescriptions was the responsibility of the compounders and the others who worked under his instructions to package the therapies on a hierarchical scale: 'There is one man whose special duty is washing bottles etc., another acts as an apprentice to the compounder … working pills masses, pounding roots, etc.'[15] Seasoned British pharmacists would claim that young British ('White') men were ill-served by arriving as apprentices in India, 'From his earliest days all his work is done by native, … he gets no practical experience in the rudiments, learns the business in a superficial way, and would not be fit, when three years in the business, to take the place of a six months' apprentice at home'.[16] Generally, the (British) pharmacist's profession was, if not ceremonial, at least a supervisory one, offering opportunities to the compounders to enhance their meagre formal knowledge with the expertise that came from the intense everyday work of mixing and preparing therapies. This was true in the private British-Indian manufacturing units as well as in the GMS workshops and continued well into the 1930s. A British pharmacist on a temporary commission in charge of the Government Medical Store in Madras during the war wrote of his Indian subordinates:

> The staff of the laboratory were chiefly native. It was a strange sight to see brown-skinned natives, all but naked, their foreheads smeared with caste-marks, attending the tablet-machines, or presiding over the stills where sp. aether was being made. They were skilful at their work, though I doubt they understood the meaning of the various operations in which they were engaged. Some had a smattering of English, but the majority spoke Tamil or Telugu.[17]

Historians have established that industrial/imperial Europeans were convinced that the 'natives' in non-European societies who worked in their laboratories or hospitals in technical roles could be taught to use scientific tools but were incapable of understanding or formulating scientific knowledge.[18] Medical research and supervisory roles were held by British medical officials in colonial India once the IMS allowed a greater number of Indians into its ranks after the Great War.

Within the RAMC, the lower-ranked regimental apothecaries' assistants were 'Eurasian'; a term originally used for the Portuguese and then more generally for mixed-race men who served above the ranks of Indian compounders, porters, and other menial workers. The large British-owned medical stores in the cities similarly employed 'Eurasians' as pharmacists' assistants. They also employed numerous Indian compounders. Some among the compounders acquired a thorough knowledge of materia medica and acquired skills on the job that might have all but equalled or even surpassed a young British pharmacist's whose knowledge tended to be formalised and whose skills were untested in a working conditions. In 1908, an indignant letter-writer complained in the London-based *Chemist and Druggist* that many qualified young British pharmacists were paid too little by the large commercial British-owned pharmacies in India and that their wages (around Rs 250/-) were only just higher than what 'native compounders' were paid.[19] Another correspondent responded to point out that the wages paid out to the non-British were exaggerated and that the Eurasians and native compounders actually did all the work at the pharmacy:

> There are about 2 per cent [Eurasians] who get so far as Rs 100 or a little more; but … these are really excellent workmen, who practically do all the work, while the English chemists go for their meals, baths, and afternoon naps in many instances. The latter luxury is never by any chance allowed to natives and Eurasians, even when they have been up almost half the night on night-duty in places like Bombay. … In places like Bombay whatever work is done after shop-hours is, as a rule, done by the native or Eurasian compounders, and not by English chemists. This is my experience, and I have been in this business over twenty years in three different places.[20]

The supervisory role adopted by young British pharmacists at the large institutions offered the Eurasian overseers and Indian compounders some flexibility with medical preparations as well as the opportunity to dispense medical advice on everyday care. After a few years of service at a military dispensary or any British commercial retailer, a Eurasian or Indian compounder could set himself up with a medical practice in a 'bazaar' pharmacy. In 1882, the Allahabad Medical Society pronounced a resolution against a Eurasian apothecary who had a lively medical practice and supplied a patient with a bottle of medicine prepared by himself, on the label of which he was described as 'Dr' and 'Surgeon'. Of course, it was not illegal to practise medicine although the description of 'Dr' could be challenged, so all the Society could do was resolve to warn him 'to refrain against such practices'.[21] The London-based trade journal *Chemist and Druggist* often published the news each time Eurasian compounders employed by British-Indian pharmacies were implicated in pilfering off supplies to bazaar pharmacists from their own stocks.[22]

The professional conflicts in India's medical praxis, therefore, were not simply between the qualified and the unqualified pharmacists but ranged across occupations engaged in producing and dispensing medicines as well as prescribing and marketing them. Medical practice in British India was served by multiple layers of dispensers that provided the 'prescription trade':

> There are a great many native doctors who have a diploma from some Indian native university, who can speak and write English, and have considerable practice. Then there are the apothecaries, who are employed by the Government in every station to take charge of the station dispensary and practice among the Government clerks, such service being given to them free, while the apothecary draws an income also from the tradespeople, many of whom employ him. The European doctors are all army surgeons, who are appointed civil surgeons in the different European stations. Besides drawing his army pay he enjoys a large income from his practice … From these different practitioners there comes a large prescription business and sale of surgical appliances etc.[23]

The points of competition and conflict between the professions of pharmacist and 'doctor' or druggist and 'compounder' occurred in both the content and form of the therapies as well as in the means of delivering them to the consumer. The first range of conflicts occurred between ex-military apothecaries who retired from the army and often established 'medical halls' (retail medical stores) in cantonments and hill stations where substantial numbers of British families resided. But they competed often against the odds, with the established European manufacturers/distributors claiming most of the customers. Therefore, they often also practised as 'doctors' in their own dispensaries. By the turn of the nineteenth century, their private practice was rivalled by emergent Indian medical professionals, many of whom had some prior experience in the subordinate services of the Indian army's medical branch.

The Indian pharmacists appointed in subordinate positions in the Indian army (the dispensaries and staff at the RAMC and the Indian army were entirely distinct) were often indistinguishable from the graduates of Indian medical colleges who practised independently, i.e., were not in government service. The Indian apothecaries in the Indian army were either former ward boys promoted by their regimental surgeons or 'sons of petty tradesmen'.[24] They signed bonds of service for five years in the Indian army as a condition of obtaining two years of training in pharmacy, materia medica, some medical knowledge, and employment in the army. As a retired British medical officer pointed out disdainfully:

> They start as doctors and chemists in the native bazaars, where there is a wide scope for counter-prescribing. They write themselves very large – "Doctor Cham Ram and Co., chemists and apothec" – and as they know how minor ailments should be treated, they often make a lot of money. I know of one retired native pharmacist who has a fine well-stocked chemists' shop in a certain bazaar and does an enormous practice as a doctor as well. His fees are only the equivalent of a shilling or so, but he is now a rich man. He even attends the poorer class of Europeans and has a great vogue amongst sergeants' wives and people of that ilk.[25]

With no specialised diploma or degree in pharmacy available in India, nor any legal bar to practising medicine, the professional lines were not demarcated. Meanwhile, most pharmacies including the prestigious British importers/wholesalers had doctors attached to their retail stores. Doctors in private practice generally found it a useful perk to have consulting rooms attached to a pharmaceutical retailer. The retailers in turn benefitted from the custom of the concerned patients and if the doctor were a reputed one, the collaboration was lucrative. It did not seem to offend professional sensibilities or any informal trading standards, British or Indian. Sir George Watt, the famous government botanist and author of several volumes on the economic botany of British India, reminisced that it was standard practice in the late nineteenth century:

> All important pharmacy establishments in India are dispensaries as well. There is a doctor attached to each of them, and he sits in an adjoining room examining patients and prescribing for them, and his fee is met by the price of the medicine supplied. That is the condition in every one of the great English pharmacists throughout India.[26]

In fact, 'private' or 'independent' practitioners of scientific medicine were much more exercised at the medical advertisements that proliferated British India; in print, on flyers distributed in public spaces, and even on the occasional wall poster or signboard. Most medical practitioners dispensed medical therapies along with medical advice from their consulting rooms, which also functioned as retail medical stores. The better-known and more enterprising vaids and hakims, as well as doctors, manufactured and offered their proprietary remedies for sale along with standard therapeutic preparations. In this sense, consultations provided by doctors within specific medical stores did not appear unusual or unethical. The services and the skills of the doctor and the pharmacist, therefore, easily resided in the same individuals who may or may not have acquired a full medical diploma or degree. 'Unqualified' doctors, including British or Eurasian pharmacists, could practice medicine in the bazaars and advertise their cures openly. An aggrieved correspondent to the *Medical Reporter* pointed out that:

> The *Indian Medical Gazette* has been shocked by the advertisement of an Indian quack, and yet our local papers are well stocked with similar advertisements from English quacks. I enclose you an advertisement ... He not only advertises his name openly, and his medicines for nameless diseases, but he fearlessly advertises that he is a Member of the Calcutta Medical Society, and nothing has been done apparently.[27]

From the 1870s, students of medicine in Bombay, Madras, and Calcutta attended one or two courses on pharmacology or materia medica. Inevitably, as the numbers of qualified Indian doctors proliferated in the twentieth century, they clashed with dispensing chemists. In the 1940s, a provincial doctor enquired of 'holders of Diploma of Pharmacy': 'Does he realise that the profession of pharmacy primarily exists to cater to the needs of a medical man and therefore the medical man is perfectly within the bounds in expecting from or insisting on, dictation to the pharmacist?'[28]

Nor was this a late colonial phenomenon. By 1905, recently qualified Indian doctors in private practice felt their livelihood and social status diminish. The profession appeared overcrowded in the cities, and Indian doctors felt that their hard-won qualifications were not respected by the public and were damaged by compounders and heterodox and eclectic practitioners of scientific medicine. The *Indian Medical Record*, representing Indian medical graduates in official and in private practice, editorialised darkly:

> In the name of common sense how can a common clerk parade himself as a physician and one able to take upon himself the honorous [*sic*] and responsible duties of a sick-bed, and yet this is exactly what is taking place; everybody and anybody to-day is a Homeopath and electropath or hypnotist, thanks to the erratic and abusive practices of these over liberal so-called scientific institutes … There are hundreds of dispensaries in Calcutta in many of which proprietors and compounders pose and ape the part of doctors, and make it a part of their business to be in secret antagonism to all regular physicians.[29]

The occupation of 'chemist and druggist' was fragmented and included everyone from unlettered bulk raw drug traders to established British manufacturers/importers. The occupation of 'compounder', therefore, encompassed multiple levels of skills and provided a range of services to the medical consumer in colonial India. A range of published materia medica or informal pharmacopeia and manuals or handbooks served to provide general guidance on making up therapies for a spectrum of illnesses and injuries. When an Indian doctor employed in the provincial subordinate medical services published a 'Dispensers' Handbook' in 1915, it included 'a useful chapter on Latin phrases and abbreviations used in writing prescriptions, a table of Latin numerals, a chapter on incompatibilities, and some tests for urine'.[30] The *IMG* endorsed it and suggested that it would be an invaluable tool for Indian compounders. In 1931, the Sind Medical Union, whose members were mostly Indian graduates of medical schools who practised privately, passed a resolution to prohibit 'unqualified allopathic practitioners' from practising as 'qualified allopathic practitioners, as 'there is a large and rapidly growing number of totally unqualified persons, chiefly of the class of ex-compounders, posing as allopathic practitioners'.[31] It is evident that the compounder continued to be indispensable in the medical market well into the 1930s. In 1931, the Drugs Enquiry Committee reported that:

> There is no organized and self-contained profession of pharmacy in India in the sense in which it exists in other parts of the world … is represented by a set of people known as compounders whose status, functions and duties are ill-defined and improperly understood. They carry

> on the compounding, dispensing and selling of drugs and chemicals from day to day. They handle drugs and poisons with the utmost ease and freedom and in many cases in ignorance of their properties and potency. They also, do work as dressers and laboratory assistants in some of the hospitals and dispensaries. Anesthetists and operation assistants are sometimes drawn from their ranks … In some· places, they pose as physicians and surgeons and acquire a position and income by no means inglorious or negligible. In respect of qualifications … they have little or none to boast of. Their standard of education is low and not much is expected of them by way of professional training.[32]

The lack of formal or scientific training in chemistry or botany on the part of the compounders was acceptable within the trade as much as the different variations of potency and quality of drugs themselves. As we have seen in chapter 5, differences in potencies and content of medical therapies differed from one retail store to another. By the 1900s, there was both an intense demand and advertising for medical therapies and wide-ranging public scepticism about their contents. Despite the near-universal disdain for the compounding class, not all or even most of these digressions from the BP could be attributed to the druggist or the uneducated compounder alone. The entire chain of manufacturers and distributors could be involved in the dilution or adulteration processes. But naturally enough, in the rare cases when such adulterations could be proved in court to have harmed the medical consumer, it was the pharmacist who was identified as the culprit. In 1911, for instance, the Calcutta High Court awarded one Elvira Molinero very substantial damages of Rs 10,000 from the chemists Dinshaw Ruttonjee Kotwal for negligence because the court was convinced that the belladonna plaster supplied to the plaintiff had caused painful blisters.[33] This lent immediacy to the strident calls in the Indian media for a food and drugs act including clarity on the legal requirements for basic qualification as a pharmacist. This was supported by British manufacturers exporting to India.

Possibly because the entire compounder class was perceived to be complicit in diluting, adding substitutes or adulterants, or otherwise compromising their products and pricing, manufacturing firms in Britain were distrustful of dispensers in India. As a prominent trade journal editorialised, 'In England pharmacists look with disfavour on the dispensing doctor. For our part, we would far rather have a dispensing doctor than an incompetent pharmacist'.[34] The professional tensions between medical practitioners and compounders escalated with the expansion of the medical market in urban India. When replying to a questionnaire from the Drugs Enquiry Committee, 67.5 per cent of respondents in Punjab, 66 per cent in Calcutta, and 60.2 per cent of respondents in Upper Provinces, all from the medical professions, complained bitterly about the lack of training and skills among compounders.[35] These tensions came into sharp relief with the increasing marketing of imported and Indigenous proprietary or pre-made medicines.

Prescriptions and Proprietaries: From Compounders to Pharmacists?

The fluidity between the professional occupations of the doctor and the dispenser informed medical cultures in one significant way: it facilitated the extensive use of proprietary medicines. While the registration of degreed and diploma-holding medical practitioners was stalled until the Drugs Act of 1940, there were repeated calls from the medical profession to curb the freely available commercial proprietary and patent medicines. These proprietary medicines were packaged conveniently, with a wide price spectrum encompassing the clientele of the British-Indian pharmacies as well as the bazaar traders. As scholars have pointed out, these proprietary medicines, especially the aphrodisiacs and 'vitality tonics', closely followed cultural trends in the public sphere. Their emphases changed from promises of potency at the turn of the century to offering fantasies for a fulfilled sexual life in the mid-1930s.[36] Similarly, nationalist, Swadeshi, as well as religious motifs, and the attraction of modern, packaged medical commodities were heavily used to market proprietary medicines that flooded the medical market.[37] The proprietary medicines encroached on doctors' and the dispensers' respective authority and income as they became ever more popular.[38]

In the proprietary medicine trade, as much as in prescription medicines, there was fierce competition among the British and American or Continental firms, with large numbers of 'bazaar' firms equally in the fray. The Indian correspondent of the *Chemist and Druggist* pointed out that the size of the proprietary market was vast and hardly touched by British traders, who focussed on prescription drugs. Instead, he pointed out, this ready market is potentially vast because 'the need for the simple proprietaries in constant sale by the ordinary pharmacist … consider the teeming millions of enervated natives who swarm in the land'.[39] Recent scholarship has established that American proprietary medicines made very successful inroads into Britain as well as further in the Indian, east Asian, and Australian markets at this time.[40] Nonetheless, British proprietary medicines, which began to be listed separately after 1924, comprised about half the value of drugs and medicines imported from Britain after the Great War.[41] Immediately after the War, a British trade journal pointed out that not only the USA and Germany, but Japan was also enhancing its proprietary trade business in India 'in the same way that she has obtained such a firm hold in China'.[42] It pointed out that the market in proprietary medicines by British manufacturers could be vastly increased if they would 'establish depots of their own in Bombay and Calcutta, to carry large stocks, to advertise widely, and to cover the market with a large number of Indian travellers' and develop a mail-order clientele.[43] And, in fact, imports from Britain continued to dominate the growing proprietary medicine trade. In 1931/32, Britain contributed 47 per cent of the total proprietary drugs imported into India, with the USA at 16 per cent, Germany at 17 per cent, France at 10 per cent, and the Netherlands, Norway, and Japan comprising the rest of the imported proprietary medicines.[44] Britain's share of the proprietary medicine trade increased to 50 per cent of the total in 1937 at the expense of German exports, possibly owing to the tariff preferences of the Ottawa agreement in 1931.[45] Not only imported medicines, but almost all manufacturers of medicines in India, Indigenous or otherwise, owned branded proprietaries as well and marketed these through retail stores, agents, and mail orders.

The expansion in the proprietary medicine trade served to change the services provided by pharmacists. The tasks of preparing prescriptions were reduced and, correspondingly, the need for at least one qualified pharmacist at even the larger chemist and druggist stores was no longer necessary. A British pharmacist who had spent years in India returned 'after 46 years' for a commercial trip to Bombay and Calcutta in 1926 and found that even in the British-Indian manufacturers' retail stores such as Bathgate and Co.:

> The dispensing department is very well arranged, a large number of prescriptions being dispensed daily; they, as well as others, find a very large

> percentage of scripts contain proprietary medicines – in fact, India must be a paradise for patent-medicine advertisers; the papers are full of advertisements; and wandering through the bazaars one finds many old preparations still on sale.[46]

Although proprietary medicines such as Dover's powder or Grey's powder had long been used in everyday medical practice in India, the sale of prepared therapies marketed as patent and proprietary medicines appeared to increase substantially in the twentieth century; the value of their imports and visibility in the public sphere were substantial.[47] These prepared nostrums for every ill, whether for minor illnesses such as headaches or colds, or long-term ones including tonics for 'vigour' and cures for diseases of the liver, stomach, or lungs flooded the stocks in the bazaar medical stores and elite medical halls at the British-Indian firms. And not only in India; the ubiquity and the scandalous deceit involved in the sale of such 'secret remedies' infuriated medical practitioners in the UK and USA from the late eighteenth century. In the nineteenth century, there were concerted efforts by medical men to isolate and expose the trade in proprietary medicines as a form of quackery.[48] Historians have related these to the rising influence and corporate professionalism of the general medicine practitioners in the USA and Britain. In Britain, the professional rivalries between chemists and druggists and general practitioners found a sharp focus on the question of authority over the sale of poisons and dangerous medicines. The British Medical Association (henceforth BMA) preferred its members, the general physicians, to have the monopoly of distribution through prescriptions and the Royal Pharmaceutical Association (henceforth RPA) for manufacturing chemists to reserve the rights of restriction of the finished goods. The sale of proprietary medicines rose ten times from 1850 to 1901 in Britain, in which period its population merely doubled.[49] After having analysed the contents of branded proprietary remedies, the BMA published two separate volumes where it detailed their contents, revealing them to be made up from commonly available and cheap (although usually harmless) substances. As historians have pointed out, in the UK, the boundary between 'quackery' and legal medicine was fluid in the eighteenth century, gradually crystallising over the nineteenth century.[50]

The rise in the sale of proprietary medicines in England was also linked to the escalation of advertisement placing in print culture, a trajectory similar to that in India although in a different century.[51] Recent scholarly work on South Asia has pointed out the ubiquity of medical advertisements in the national and vernacular presses, affording large transnational firms and smaller, 'bazaar' manufacturers the opportunity to widely advertise their proprietary medicines.[52] Although elite IMS officials berated the flood of medical advertisements for proprietary medicines, there was little legislation to prevent it. The Government of India did enact a patent law in 1911 but there were enough loopholes for proprietary medicines to slip through its restrictions.[53]

The easy availability of proprietary medicines correspondingly made the medical dispenser's task simple. By 1939, trained and experienced pharmacists at large stores in the presidency capitals could claim that the great increase in the use of proprietary medicines correspondingly diminished profits and deskilled their profession.[54] In the late colonial years, the ubiquity of proprietary medicines was reflected in the fact that almost two-thirds of medicines dispensed at large medical stores were proprietary and pre-packaged therapies. This sharpened the competition between the European chemists and druggists and the 'bazaar' medical stores: 'these patent medicines can be had at competitive prices from any shop in the bazaar'.[55] It also further enabled an easier practise of medicine on the part of Western as well as Indigenous medical practitioners. A British-Indian pharmaceutical chemist-manufacturer in Lahore deposed to the Drugs Enquiry Committee in 1930 that 'compounders in the Punjab … have very little education … I have employed compounders who have held responsible positions in Government hospitals and found I had to train them as beginners'.[56]

Conclusion: The Compounder and the Fluid Medical Market

The professional boundary between the druggist and the doctor or even the formal distinction prevalent in contemporary Britain between the manufacturing chemists and the chemist and druggist did not emerge with the expansion of the medical market and diversification in the medical cultures. The medical culture accommodated qualified pharmacists, untrained compounders, dispensing doctors, and prescribing druggists with similar flexibility with which it countenanced Indigenous and imported therapies of varying potencies and standards of purity. It is at the site of medical praxis, of preparation of therapies, their marketing in local and regional presses, and sale to medical consumers that the eclecticism of medicine in colonial India was manifest. The DEC pointed out in 1931, for instance, how the doctors themselves dispensed medicines with their compounders, taking care to conceal from the public their prescriptions and in the process depriving chemist and druggist stores of retail trade in Madras:

> In Madras private medical practitioners … Usually … dispense their own prescriptions … they do not charge for professional services but make an inclusive charge when charging for medicine. Some of them. to ensure that the prescriptions are dispensed in their own establishments and are in the habit of using code words for the drugs known only to the practitioner and his compounder.[57]

In this context, the compounder not only fit within the eclectic medical market, but he was also a product of the eclectic market. Any attempt to streamline the training and qualification of pharmacists would be bound to legislation on standardized drug regulations and monitoring. Compounders often worked on the margins of the medical market and personified the fluidity between Indigenous and scientific therapies, or the slippage of boundaries between the roles of the medical practitioner and the medical dispenser.[58] In 1911, for instance, district officials in the Malabar districts responded to government enquiries about Indigenous medical institutions by pointing out that the two well-run Ayurvedic hospitals in Malabar employed 'qualified' compounders who could also dispense B.P. prescriptions.[59] With the wide and varying roles that compounders fulfilled, their social status differed greatly even without taking the always-present racial and caste hierarchies into account. When the Director General of the IMS published a 'medical review' to highlight the expansion of medical institutions and infrastructure in British India in 1938, he showed that eligibility for the rudimentary training of compounders available in Indian provinces was varied but universally low. In some provinces, entrants into the compounders' training courses (lasting a few months) required only the completion of a primary school education.[60] Meanwhile, lapses in the quality of medicines in government hospitals continued to be attributed to the 'inaccurate dispensing and carelessness' of the compounders rather than on their qualified superior officials or on the supply of the raw drug itself.[61] In 1940, R.N. Chopra who had chaired the Drugs Enquiry Committee repeated his scathing indictment of the compounder's profession and its connection with drug adulteration in India:

> The profession of pharmacy here is represented by a class of people called, 'compounders', whose status, functions and duties are ill defined … They … dispense medicines including the most potent preparations and deadly poisons in many cases in complete ignorance of their properties and potency. They also work as dressers, laboratory and hospital assistants, anaesthetists, operation assistants and as male nurses in many mofussil hospitals and dispensaries. They are often called upon to undertake the duties of the medical officer … and usually pass as 'doctors' before the lay public. Many of them carry a stethoscope in their pockets and frequently give intravenous injections.[62]

When the first pharmaceutical associations were formed in Calcutta and Bombay after the Great War, these involved large pharmaceutical manufacturers/distributors, including both British-owned and wholly Indian enterprises. These were trade associations rather than a professional body of pharmacists or dispensing chemists. Briefly, after the Great War, they organised themselves and ran a collective campaign to protect their interests. Their concerns included the unfavourable rise in exchange rates between the pound and the rupee, the demands for a more modern excise system that excluded alcohol-based medical therapies from paying taxes on the alcohol content of their commodities, and more equitable railway freights. The Pharmaceutical Associations in the Bengal and Bombay Presidencies, therefore, represented the commercial interests of the large manufacturing firms and articulated their specific concerns to the government and occasionally in public.

As far as the dispensing chemists and compounders of varied qualifications and experience were concerned, they did not have a collective association or a trade journal to offer their perspectives and protect their interests. Unlike Indian doctors who qualified in Indian medical colleges and joined the subordinate medical services, the thousands of compounders who dispensed prescriptions in medical stores had no professional regulations or any way of generating collective action. Some of the better-paid Indian druggists in southern India took a few courses on pharmacy at the Madras Medical College, but these did not amount to a government-recognised full diploma.[63] The DEC recommended full training for pharmacists at medical colleges. It was not until 1937 that a college of pharmacy was established in Vizagapatnam, and in that year the Benares Hindu University began a full diploma in pharmacy, with Punjab following soon with a similar diploma.[64] The Drugs Acts of 1944 legislated for a streamlined syllabus in medical colleges and went on to abolish all training of provincial 'licensed medical practitioners' and stipulated a full five-year training programme (Bachelor of Medicine and Bachelor of Surgery) for all doctors practising Western medicine. This facilitated the formal training of pharmacists. The Pharmacy Act (1948) also stipulated a Pharmacy Council of India as the governing body for the entire profession and for regulating the examination boards in each administrative province. Both diplomas (two years of formal study) and degrees (three years of formal study) in pharmacy were initiated in medical colleges once the Pharmacy Council of India was established only in the independent nation-state in 1949, with state councils to be established regionally at a later time.

In 1954, the much-awaited Pharmaceutical Committee report pointed out that despite the regulation of the Pharmacy Act most chemists and druggists' stores employed compounders of uncertain training and uneven experience: 'The profession of pharmacy in this country is mostly represented by a set of people known as compounders, whose status, functions and duties are ill-defined and improperly understood. Their pharmaceutical education is deplorably inadequate and the majority of them employed in the trade have had none at all'.[65] The role of the compounder, therefore, remained within the interstices of professionalisation and the triumph of biomedicine in the post-independence era. By 1963, eleven institutions offered a diploma or degree in pharmacy, with the graduate degree holders generally employed with manufacturing chemists and diploma holders as medical dispensers in hospitals and medical stores.[66] Therefore, the institutionalisation of formal pharmacy education occurred slowly; the pharmacist replaced the compounder only in the well-established metropolitan retail stores. Somewhat like the eclectic medicines sold over the counter, the dispensers remained heterogeneous.

7

Drugs for the Nation

This chapter explores why self-sufficiency in synthetic drugs became the paradigm of drug policy in the early years of the postcolonial nation-state. Scholarly discussions on independent India's successful pharmaceutical industries (and self-sufficiency in medicines) tend to focus on the Patent Act of 1970.[1] This was when the Government of India enabled the patent of the process but not of the product so that Indian firms could manufacture generic drugs. The limitation of foreign direct investment to 49 per cent further strengthened Indian enterprise in pharmaceuticals. The Indian pharmaceutical industry and its dependence on the manufacture of generic drugs, and the manufacturing sector and government's struggles with intellectual property rights agreements, tend to dominate contemporary discourse on the Indian pharmaceutical industry.

As we have seen so far, the issues of self-sufficiency in medicines and the availability of cheap and efficacious drugs for all were politically potent and explicit in colonial India and nationalist discourse. The problems of adulteration and standardization, questions around import substitution, and the largely unregulated cultures of dispensing medicines were all premised on the need to provide cheap and efficacious drugs for people.

The postcolonial state carried the mandate of self-sufficiency in food and medicines through the Nehruvian model of protectionist industrialism and scientific planning. Historians have offered insights into science policy and planning in Nehruvian India that can explain policies and trends in making and marketing medicines in the post-independence years. As the architect of modern India and the politician who invited scientists to participate in the politics of nation building, Nehru enabled the new nation-state to posit science as both Indigenous and emancipatory. This anticipated the creation of both an enlightened postcolonial citizenry and a centralised government that planned scientific progress through state initiatives and planning.[2] Historiographical debates have reflected on the nature of the colonial and the nation-state's respective commitments to scientific research and industrial planning, the scholarly consensus being that scientific industrialism was rhetorically privileged but severely underfunded in late colonial India.[3]

This chapter will, therefore, examine how medicines continued to be made and marketed in the new nation-state. This is not to re-evaluate the historiographical consensus on Nehruvian science or revisit the debate on state support for Indian industry. Instead, this chapter will demonstrate how the state became the chief arbitrator in this culture of disparate remedies. Indian medicine manufacturing units either benefited from state support or were entirely state owned in the post-independence era, and the subsequent expansion of private production of pharmaceuticals did so in the contexts of political and ideological support for self-sufficiency and affordable medicines for all citizens. It will finally identify how the Indigenous and Western medical markets acquired distinct identities even while the latter was being marginalised in mainstream medical praxis and by the Indian state.

Postcolonial Conundrums: Self-Sufficiency and the Biomedicine Gap

The period after 1945 was one of dominance for biomedicine. In Britain, on the Continent, and in the USA, the medical establishment and the state favoured biomedical solutions to complex diseases. Most spectacularly visible in the successful treatment of bacterial infections and used and perfected in military medicine for the treatment of wounds were sulpha drugs and antibiotics, which fuelled dreams of magic bullets and cure for disease.[4] As several ancient, terrifying, infectious illnesses could finally be diminished, medical institutions in industrialised nation-states adopted them enthusiastically.

Therefore, although the UK, France, and the USA had different models for public health and medical research and differing relationships between medical research, clinical experiments, and public health, the use of sulpha drugs and antibiotic treatment for the cure of infectious diseases became a common factor in their medical regimes. Despite hesitations and the lingering presence of alternative medical viewpoints, in the post-Second-World-War era, all roads appeared to point towards biomedical solutions in public health.[5] Although they were never entirely banished, especially in the UK, older sanitarian models of epidemic control became marginalized. The use of sulpha drugs and penicillin changed the framework of curative medicine and strengthened the global power of pharmaceutical companies based in the Western world. In turn, drugs derived from botanical and mineral materials dwindled in significance. One of the most visible instances of the turn towards synthetic drugs was mepacrine, and later paludrine, the synthetic antimalarials that were substituted for quinine and proved crucial to the Allies' victories on the Eastern Front.[6] Synthetic vitamins and hormonal drugs were in circulation in the colonial medical markets globally; in the Second World War, IMS officials were able to witness first-hand how penicillin and sulpha drugs could transform curative medicine in the field hospitals.

As we have seen in previous chapters, the fledgling pharmaceutical industry had consistently demanded government support in taxation, procurement policy, and for establishing technological and pedagogical infrastructure. The Indian Industrial Commission's report (1918) had fallen short of nationalist demands for protectionism to national industry.[7] Moreover, its recommendation for an Indian Chemical Service to enable research and training for heavy and fine chemical manufacturing, including pharmaceuticals, was ignored by the Government of India. After 1930, when the government finally appointed a Tariffs Board, it granted limited and temporary protection to seven industries including cotton textiles, steel, sericulture, paper, and sugar, but not to Indigenous drugs or medicines. As we have seen in chapter 4, after 1920, the reformulated Stores Department was directed to procure supplies from India whenever possible, but this barely changed the volume of imported medicines or drugs purchased by the government.

The DEC's report proposed structural changes and substantial pecuniary and administrative support from the government to facilitate drug manufacture and a market closely monitored by the government. The DEC published its report in 1931 and recommended comprehensive drug legislation and scientific and official infrastructure for monitoring compliance. The infrastructure was needed to establish central and provincial drug laboratories to test, assay, and implement drug standardisation. The government established a central drug laboratory after some delay. Despite the limited devolution of power after 1920, most provincial governments argued that they did not have the resources to maintain a drug laboratory and requested that the central government take responsibility for this. The Drugs Bill 1940 and Pharmacy Bill 1944 legislated for standardisation and professionalisation of pharmacy. Although questions remained about the precise nature of the formal training that pharmacists would receive, the inadequacy of provisions for their training, and so on, this settled the course of training for pharmacy and dispensing. Once the central drug testing laboratories and vaccines were established in 1937, the remit of which included medicines as well as vaccines and sera, the emphasis in public discourse and government policy shifted from the quality/content of medicine to self-sufficiency in medicines and drugs. Therefore, the post-independence narrative of drug production in India is dominated by the lure of self-sufficiency and import substitution, but of antibiotics and synthetic drugs.

There were two distinct contexts for this shift. The first was the Indian National Congress and its National Planning Committee (NPC). The policy documents laid out the vision for the emergent nation-state, to be founded on welfare for all (or development, to use the expert technical term) through large-scale industrialism. It was a seminal moment and represented the first significant move that would culminate in the scientific industrialism that characterised the Nehruvian postcolonial state. The resignation of the provincial Congress ministries in 1939 and the political repression unleashed by the colonial government in its death throes resulted in the dissolution of the NPC by 1940. The NPC, however, secured that doubts about large-scale industrialisation on the part of Gandhians were firmly marginalised. Instead, scientific experts created plans for the economic (and, thereby, political) future of the postcolonial state.[8]

The British government entirely ignored the NPC. Sovereign neglect, however, did not withstand the pressures of the Second World War. The commencement of the War brought into sharp relief the gaps in medical provision within the Indian subcontinent just as it had done in the First World War, and with greater urgency. The Second World War advanced Indian industry and pharmaceutical products and surgical instruments were some of its largest beneficiaries, in the Indian continent as well as in the USA, Germany, Japan, and the UK. All the trends previously discussed – institutes to test the standard of drugs, vaccines, and sera; frantic research for import substitutions and research on the large-scale cultivation of drugs both of Indian and foreign origin within India; the emphasis on local manufacture of vitamins and hormones through local biological materials; a renewed interest in systematising Indigenous medicine; legislation to curb the worst excesses of the patent-medicine industry; professionalization of medical practice and pharmacy – all were invested in a compelling topicality and experienced incremental expansion.

The War and the Pharmaceutical Industry

In 1938, the DGIMS published an overview of the curative institutions and the state of (Western) medical practice and training in India in the aftermath of the devolution of power and further provincialisation of health services in 1937, except for control over port quarantine and a few premier research institutes.[9] His report emphasised the acute shortage of qualified doctors in India; on average there was one doctor for every 10,000 people in India. The next comprehensive all-India survey of the state of medical care was published on the eve of independence: the Government of India's Health Survey and Development (Bhore) Commission's report.[10] It observed in painful detail the abysmal death and morbidity rates from disease and the lack of medical care among the vast majority of the Indian population. Its most significant proposal was to establish primary health centres and make these the centre of preventive and curative health programmes in rural India. Much of the soul-searching about the state's role in public health in newly independent India has referred to the report. Visions for public health in the postcolonial state have produced templates that address the infrastructural shortcomings and have generated a developmental model of public health.[11]

The other significant factor that informed government policy on medical infrastructure and resources was the Second World War. Most resources, material or human, made their way to the war effort, causing scarcity. The opening of the Eastern Front drained money, men, livestock, food, and medicine from the entire Indian subcontinent.[12] The Quit India Movement, begun by the Congress in 1942, galvanised nationalist sentiments, and highlighted that much of the Indian population begrudged the British their very presence in India and resented the huge outflow of resources that the war had occasioned. In the chaos of the war and expectations of a Japanese invasion into mainland India proper, scarcities of basic commodities of food, cloth, and medicine proliferated, as did speculation and hoarding, creating yet further scarcity and higher prices.[13] Just like it had done in the Great War but in a greatly enhanced form, the Second World War both exposed the over-dependence on imported drugs and therapeutics and generated a huge leap in their production by Indian manufacturers. Until 1941, private distributors and importers were content with the supply from Europe. The editorial of the leading trade journal in India pointed out that:

> Soon after the war broke out most of the business firms dealing in drugs were apprehensive ... But experience has since shown that there is no difficulty in the importation of drugs both from Great Britain and America, sufficient to supply the needs of this country. Efficient substitutes for some of the specialities which had to be imported from Germany are also procurable from other countries ... [at] certain amount of delay and extra cost ... Thanks to the action taken up by various local governments there has been no appreciable profiteering in drugs and most of the drugs are procurable in the market at reasonable prices.[14]

This early optimism withered as the war escalated in Europe and supplies to India were disrupted and practically dried up. Indian drug and surgical instrument manufacturers hastily consolidated themselves into a trade association, much as they had during the Great War. The government, military, and commerce departments were involved. Realising that imports would eventually stop entirely, the Government of India supervised the acceleration of the production of sera, summoned drug manufacturers for information on their existing capacity, discussed how to extend the production of drugs by both the GMS and the private manufacturers, and made arrangements to buy cinchona in bulk from the Dutch conglomerates.[15] By 1942, Indian manufacturers had diversified their products and intensified the volume of production, with the support of the GMS.[16] Later in that year, the DGIMS's office declared that,

'Two hundred and ninety two drugs and … other items of medical supplies formerly imported are now being manufactured by Indian drug manufacturers or Government medical-depot factories'[17]. The government declared that these drugs were now transferred to the Indigenous list; of the 292 drugs now manufactured in India, twenty-eight were available in plentiful supplies, enough to be exported as well as used within India.[18] The newly instituted association liaised regularly with the DGIMS's office for support towards facilitating imports of raw materials such as quinine and other chemicals to help diversify and extend the products of the drug industry. Unsurprisingly, most medicine produced by Indian manufacturers was used by the Indian army, and normal supplies for everyone else were reduced greatly. The trade association, which included manufacturers who imported bulk drugs for processing as well as importers and distributors, began to ration their products to private customers, hospitals, and dispensaries. Acutely aware of discontent due to their enforced rationing, the trade association wrote an unprecedented open letter to the elite medical practitioners explaining their predicament, denying their responsibility for the speculative rise in drug prices, and appealing to medical associations to help lobby the government to expedite drug imports:

> The aim is to distribute all supplies … as evenly and to as many … patrons as possible, and … the necessity for what may appear to be drastic rationing on their part when small supplies become available from time to time. In this connection the Medical Profession will also appreciate the fact that despite only limited stocks available for distribution, the main distributors have not put up prices beyond legitimate limits, and are in no way responsible for the unprecedented speculative trend of the present-day drug market.
>
> … My committee therefore wishes that the leading Medical Associations should use their influence in persuading the principal authorities concerned in Import Trade Control … to facilitate an adequate supply of at least essential medicines which are required for the civil population.[19]

Therefore, during the Second World War, medicine or drugs required for the private market or even for civil hospitals and dispensaries mostly relied on local production. The dedicated research conducted by Ram Nath Chopra and his associates at the CSTM over the previous two decades had provided the foundation for the legitimation of the two hundred-odd drugs produced in India. Between 1927 and 1940, at his laboratory in the CSTM, Chopra and his colleagues had painstakingly collected, analysed, and identified the active components of hundreds of drugs. These were published in medical and scientific journals regularly. The drugs, some of common origin and plentiful in supply, once validated by scientific investigation were intended for cultivation on a large scale wherever possible. And indeed, besides cinchona and opium (the only systematic medicinal cultivation in India until then), digitalis, nux vomica (strychnine), belladonna, and Indian substitutes for ipecacuanha were all examined, experimented upon, and pronounced as suitable for mass production in India. Drugs derived from botanical materials – ephedra, belladonna, artemisia – were cultivated in the Indian subcontinent and although much more could be done to extend their cultivation, these were used to manufacture drugs within India. In 1940, Chopra pointed out to an assembly of the newly formed association of pharmaceutical manufacturers that 'nearly three-fourths of the drugs mentioned in the British and other pharmacopeias grow here in a state of nature or have been cultivated', and that 'where the pharmacopeial species do not grow, allied species are available which may be used as substitutes'.[20] As Chopra noted, the bottlenecks remained in the lack of availability of heavy chemicals such as sulphuric acid, iodine, and bromine, which were essential to the manufacturing process for organic drugs, and were mostly imported at that time. Therefore, the manufacture of medicine was limited to some galenicals, essential oils (sandalwood, clove, rose), oils (linseed, almond), a limited number of glandular and hormonal products (vitamins, insulin), and sera and vaccines. It was estimated just before the war that the volume of production of medicines within India comprised roughly a third of the total volume of imports of medicines into India. The sera and vaccines were produced mostly at the government research centre at the Haffkine Institute, with the exception of one firm, Bengal Immunity, that had been established in 1919 and continued to research and produce vaccines and sera during the Second World War and beyond.[21] However, private pharmaceutical firms focussed on either manufacturing galenicals or on importing bulk drugs from foreign firms and producing synthetic drugs from these.[22] Indian medical and scientific officials such as Lt. Colonel S.S. Sokhey, then director of the Haffkine Institute in Bombay, or R.N Chopra, himself, rued the inadequacy of Indian drug manufacturers who seldom invested in research to develop new drugs and 'had resorted to mere compounding, mostly out of imported pharmaceuticals'.[23]

Despite heated debates and contrary opinions on how to impose a standard of quality on drugs, both a drug and a pharmacy bill passed through the legislature, and by 1944, India finally had a drugs act. Although the institutionalisation of standardisation, as well as the professionalisation of pharmacy, remained incomplete, once the legislation was secured, universities introduced courses on pharmacy and manufacturers standardised their commodities and made the ingredients transparent.

The Marginalisation of Botanical and Mineral Drugs

The war raised yet again the government and the medical communities' focus on using Indigenous drugs to manufacture therapeutic products in India. The desire for Indigenous drugs was simply a pragmatic one – to replace expensive and scarce imported drugs – and this urgency was naturally heightened during times of crisis. However, after the Second World War, Indigenous drugs were once again relegated to relative obscurity. Apart from the small quantities that could be processed through the scientific idiom of their active principles, the cultivated and known medicinal plants such as cinchona or digitalis were demonstrably of a relatively low potency. This rendered their large-scale production uneconomic and unsustainable in the long term.

More significantly, botanical drugs, even identifiable and potent ones, paled in significance to the enchantment of the newly emerged sulpha drugs and antibiotics. In the post-war years, the elite in the Indian medical community increased the use and awareness of sulpha drugs and, later, of antibiotics.

> It is evident then that, under such conditions, factors other than cure rates must enter into the consideration of the public health measures to be adopted. The private physician is not necessarily so limited in his management of patients financially able to pay for treatment, since his responsibility and services may be more narrowly confined to the circle

> of his clientele. Nevertheless, the use of any penicillin-schedule in underdeveloped areas, such as are found in India, must be based on the availability of the drug. Penicillin is not yet made commercially in these countries, and must therefore be imported and paid for from the 'hard currency' reserves of the governments. Thus, the choice of therapeutic schedules in public health work must be based upon what is practical for the country and not upon what is considered ideal in the USA.[24]

The WHO's initial medical aid to South Asia focussed on targeted programmes for specific diseases with the new sulpha drugs and antibiotics and trained local medical personnel to use them as well.[25] Moreover, the IMS had used antibiotics during the Second World War extensively in military medicine and disseminated clinical experiences of these in medical journals. The use of sulpha drugs and antibiotics extended into private medical practice as well, in so far as these were available for use for non-military purposes. In a typhus epidemic in Calcutta in 1949, for instance, a medical official reported that:

> Most patients had expectant therapy, alkaline mixture, imperial drink, gargles, linctus, vitamins, sedatives, cardiac stimulants, etc., having been used as required. A number of patients had penicillin therapy either empirically before the diagnosis was made but without any effect, or for secondary complications ... The recently discovered antibiotics Chloromycetin and aureomycin which had been found to be specific against typhus fever could not be procured.[26]

Treating epidemic disease, even in instances of both the poverty of the sick and the scarcity of penicillin or sulpha drugs, had firmly shifted to the use of these new wonder drugs in the early 1950s, and these trends were reflected in the pharmacopeia. The *Indian Medical Gazette* pointed out in 1953 that the just published BPa had dropped 148 single drugs (monograph), added 115, and excluded nineteen vegetable drugs. The editorial pointed out that 'the additions are in keeping with the advices in chemotherapy and antibiotics' and appealed for other standard works to include these supposedly obsolete drugs because they were needed and used in India.[27] The political economy of medicine, therefore, now largely rested on the import, distribution, and

Indigenous production of the antibiotics themselves. In public discourse and everyday medical praxis, the use of sulpha drugs and antibiotics assumed the status of a primacy a priory. [28]

Meanwhile, ten years after the publication of Bradfield's report, the National Planning Commission's health sub-committee presented its long-delayed report. The sub-committee, chaired by S.S. Sokhey, formerly in charge of the Haffkine's Institute, was to define the postcolonial state's priorities and strategies in public health and curative medicine. The report emphasised the need for self-sufficiency in drugs for India. However, it also noted that the progress in research on Indian materia medica had served to eliminate several drugs from the modern Indian Pharmacopeia:

> It is well to remember that, until recent times, the pharmacopoeia of all countries were uncritical compilations of all sorts of drugs,- and India is no exception, except that the 'unofficial' pharmacopoeia of India and its systems of medicine have not been adequately revised for centuries. With the development of the scientific methods of assessing pharmacological and therapeutic value of drugs, all the pharmaco-poeias [*sic*] have been steadily discarding larger and larger number of these drugs at each revision, as the tests have shown them to be of no value.[29]

Although the aims of self-sufficiency in drugs and medicines remained and were strengthened in nationalist discourse and government planning and policy, the report pointed out that:

> Great advances have been made in the preparation of new drugs with specific action in given diseases. The drugs so produced are some of the greatest achievements of scientific medicine … To our mind, then, the solution of the problem of the expensiveness of the drugs is not to use inert and useless drugs, though cheap; but to produce effective needed drugs cheaply in the country.[30]

The sub-committee appointed another committee under the chairmanship of R.N. Chopra to elucidate fully how drugs and medicines could be produced in India cheaply and in enough quantities for self-sufficiency. The committee's conclusions, arrived at after consultation with the Indian Chemical Manufacturers' Association, pointed out that most synthetic and 'chemo-therapeutic' products, as well as vitamins and biological products such as sera and vaccines, could potentially be manufactured in India. It needed the government to offer protection to the industry to ensure that the manufacture of essential chemicals including sulphuric acid, benzol, petroleum ether, and starch was increased substantially, and to assure their regular imports meanwhile.[31] While not disregarding botanical drugs entirely, the report indicated priorities were changing in the direction of producing therapeutic drugs.

Moreover, of the fourteen sub-committees of the NPC, the sub-committee on the chemical industry (which had private entrepreneurs including B.D. Amin as its members) also pointed out that so far as drugs were concerned, 'Government assistance and initiative are required in establishing this industry on a sound basis. The country should be made self-sufficient'.[32]

In effect, the hoary debates on the standardization and relevance of Indigenous drugs to modern medicine became peripheral to the state and to the medical market and its consumers at this time. Instead, the debates in the first two decades of the independent nation ranged from how to achieve self-sufficiency in drugs to enabling a government-supported health service for all. Ideological and strategic policy tensions were reflected in debates on public ownership or private enterprise in drug manufacture, the role of universities or specialised research institutions in drug research, and competing models of delivering rural health services.

Self-Sufficiency and the Nation-State

Although the Second World War enabled a rapid rise in drugs production, these were limited to immediate demands and did not significantly include the expansion of the manufacture of synthetic drugs. The new government instituted several enquiries that submitted substantial reports on the state of the chemical and pharmaceutical industries and offered strategies for enhancing production. These included a panel on fine chemicals and drugs in 1948, a panel on the drug industry in 1951, and advisory within the first Planning Commission. The reports invariably emphasised how vital it was to enhance the production of synthetic drugs and antibiotics to reduce costly imports. The disagreements among the committees verged only on the specific modes of achieving these; whether to support private or public industry, where to locate the new industries, how to best consolidate existing infrastructures and to sustain the technical skills needed for large-scale industrialisation of the production of pharmaceuticals. Scientific opinion and public discourse too favoured industrialisation to facilitate self-sufficiency in drugs, although robust debates on the extent of government ownership or foreign investments needed for these prevailed. When the NPC's Health Report was published, for instance, *Current Science*, a Bangalore-based nationalist periodical, strongly approved of the government's prospective joint venture with a Swedish company to manufacture antibiotics but pointed out that Bangalore was much better suited for the industry than the proposed location in Bombay.[33] As Nasir Tyabji has shown, the new nation-state had to use Cold-War rivalries to negotiate technical and financial support, balancing the proposals of pharmaceutical giants in the USA and Sweden versus offers from the World Health Organization (WHO) and UNICEF.[34] In spite of international pressures and lobbying from within by Indian manufacturers that wished to partner with transnational firms, when the first antibiotics factory was set up in Pimpri near Poona, the WHO's offer of sharing the technology and supporting costs for the infrastructure proved more attractive to the postcolonial state.[35] The agreement was signed in 1951, and the first antibiotic factory in India, Hindustan Antibiotics Limited, was government-owned with financial and technological support from the WHO and UNICEF.[36] By the time Hindustan Antibiotics began manufacturing in 1955, the prices of synthetic drugs in India, almost all imported, were among the highest in the world. The government commissioned a separate committee to collect information and deliver recommendations for the drug and pharmaceutical industry, which submitted its report in 1954. Meanwhile, the government signed agreements with American and German firms for technological support in manufacturing various antibiotics and sulphonamides in Pimpri. The USSR helped with technology and support to plan for and build eight synthetic drug manufacturing units in Rishikesh, Hyderabad, and other locations in India between 1951 and 1959. A new state-owned company, the IDPL, was established as the umbrella firm for the manufacturing companies.

The Pharmaceuticals Enquiry (Bhatia) Committee Report (1954) acknowledged the progress made through foreign and government technological and financial support to the pharmaceutical industry. It pointed out that the Planning Commission had recently noted that:

> Higher priority should be given to the manufacture of synthetic drugs than to the manufacture of imported drugs into tablets or finished preparations for use.
>
> Whenever penultimate products and complex intermediates are used in the first instance to start the industry, efforts should be directed towards manufacturing … within the country as soon as possible.[37]

Both priorities identified by the first Planning Commission – privileging synthetic drugs over botanical/mineral drugs and the lack of access to technological know-how on the part of Indian collaborators of pharmaceutical MNCs – were revealed in clearer detail by the Bhatia Commission. Its report sharply criticised the high 'royalties' (12 to 15 per cent) charged by pharmaceutical MNCs and the blatantly unequal collaborations with Indian partners:

> Even in the case of production of essential drugs and pharmaceuticals, the agreements refer only to 'know-how' of their processing i.e., ampouling, granulating … or compounding of imported pharmaceuticals, but not to their manufacture from basic ingredients. These royalty payments … stipulated as royalty for the supply of blueprints and other engineering facilities and advice … of the foreign firm for the supply of the 'know-how'. Such huge royalties on finished products imported in bulk and only repacked in this country seem unwarranted.[38]

The Pharmaceutical Enquiry (1954) report advised increasing capacity to enable self-sufficiency in drugs and in strategic chemicals that were required for their production, including alkalies, acids, and alcohol. In the Nehruvian planning stage, the public-owned Hindustan Antibiotics Limited in Pimpri was followed by the establishment of the government-owned India Drugs and Pharmaceuticals Limited (IDPL). The IDPL set up factories to produce antibiotics and other synthetic drugs in Rishikesh and Hyderabad with aid from the USSR.[39] A British government official advised Wellcome Burroughs of London that Hindustan Antibiotics Limited had the capacity to produce nine million mega units of penicillin per annum and that the IDPL had the capacity to produce 850 tons of antibiotics annually in Hyderabad, 300 tons in Rishikesh, and had planned further expansion in units across the country.[40] In 1962, the government production of pharmaceuticals comfortably outpaced private manufactures in antibiotics and botanical drugs and was neck-and-neck in the synthetic drugs sector.

Along with the production of public-owned manufacturing units, the Pharmaceutical Enquiry report (1954) recommended that privately owned synthetic and antibiotic manufacturers, as well as those producing vitamins and hormonal therapies, be offered tariff concessions to facilitate maximum production of essential medicines. It suggested that MNCs that collaborated with Indian firms be required to manufacture basic chemicals as well as process the drugs within India instead of importing expensive chemicals or bulk drugs. B.D. Amin of Alembic Chemical Works was a member of the committee and, perhaps unsurprisingly given that he had been vocal on this issue in all public forums for decades, the report referred to restructuring the excise regime to exclude pharmaceutical manufacturers from paying excise duties for the pure alcohol used in their alcohol-based products. Overall, the Bhatia Committee pointed unambiguously towards the goal of self-sufficiency from imported pharmaceutical products. Its recommendations included strong government support for infrastructure and initiatives for the transfer of technology. The Committee pointed out that the expansion of the production of medicines would need to take place through government-owned firms as well as private ones. Therefore, although socialized medicine was out of reach, state-protected industrial production of synthetic drugs and antibiotics was considered achievable. The government's partnerships did not reduce the role of private entrepreneurship in producing medicines, nor was it expected to do so.

The Drugs Act of 1944 was to serve as the legislative bulwark against fraud in fake medicine and provide for qualified doctors, nurses, and pharmacists. Despite alternative suggestions, there was no attempt to allow licensciates (LMPS, etc.) to practise as doctors; only graduates of five-year degree programmes from authorised medical colleges were to be granted the title of doctor. Similarly, several medical colleges introduced training programmes for pharmacists and nurses in the pattern of Western industrialized nations. It

Table 7.1
Summary of manufacture of pharmaceuticals in India, 1962

	Private industry tons/annum	*GOI undertakings tons/annum*
Antibiotics	74.6	373.6
Synthetic drugs	1,719.8	1,551.0
Drugs of vegetable origin	49.6	71.4
Total	1,844.0	1,996.0

Source: Clipping from *Eastern Economist*, 2 February 1962, titled 'Pharmaceuticals: Towards Self-Sufficiency' in Mss/Eur 158/265 IOR/APAC, British Library, London.

was clear that even with the modest increase in the number of medical colleges, the doctor-patient ratio would remain abysmal in rural areas and inadequate in urban or semi-urban areas. Nonetheless, in the early 1960s, there was little attempt to train the so-called barefoot doctors in the model of the Chinese state to cater to the rural population. The Indian nation-state adopted the PHC (primary health care centres) as the principal point of contact in rural areas and many of them remained bereft of qualified physicians, nurses, and pharmacists.[41]

By the early 1960s, self-sufficiency in medicines was firmly situated within the framework of industrial production of synthetic drugs and antibiotics. Medical and official discourses as well as public opinion on medical care referenced these as essential medicines and distinct from botanical drugs. Although opium and cinchona continued to be cultivated in the older government plantations and processed into therapeutic commodities, their use too was on the wane. The distinctions between Western and non-Western medicine, so indeterminate in the medical cultures of India, became clearer and easier to articulate. With their increased prescription and use in hospitals and private practice, Western medicines became the mainstream therapies of choice. Even cash-strapped local bodies and municipal hospitals preferred to spend their meagre allocation of funds on buying antibiotics or synthetic drugs. The promise of the delivery of health care to impoverished rural areas was made on the ideal of establishing economical primary health centres (PHCs) and accelerating the volume of production of the new synthetic drugs. Indigenous medical therapies had ceased to appeal to policy makers and the public.

Indigenous Medicine in Independent India

Scholarship on contemporary Ayurveda is agreed that Ayurveda is globally successful and discusses the ways in which therapeutic, cosmetic, and food and beverages manufacturers have branded their products and captured a specific market within the multi-billion dollar 'well-being' industry. It is possible to consume Ayurvedic medicines, fruits and vegetable juices and extracts, clarified butter, and purchase dozens of cosmetic products globally today. Along with these, the older, more familiar concoctions of branded tonics, blood cleansers, hair oils, and toothpastes similarly continue to crowd the shelves in medical stores in physical and online marketplaces.

Despite the explosion in the marketability of Ayurvedic products, they occupy the position of 'alternative' or more positively, 'complementary' therapies. So far as their specific therapeutic commodities are concerned, they are usually directed towards chronic afflictions, not acute diseases. The most recognisable and long-standing Indigenous therapeutic products are Dabur's and Zandu's 'Chyavanprash', which is a health tonic, and Hamdard's 'Rooh-Afza', a beverage of rose extract and herbs. The affluence of manufacturers of Ayurvedic firms is dwarfed by the profits of pharmaceutical companies.

This trajectory was not inevitable, but the clear strategies on public health and infrastructure favoured by the postcolonial government narrowed the scope of expansion or research in Indigenous drugs. The political momentum of nationalist support for Indigenous drugs did not disappear entirely. At the time of independence, the fate of the Indigenous drug industry and its practitioners was of significance in public life. The central government commissioned R.N. Chopra to lead an investigation into how Indigenous systems of medicine, their practitioners, and institutions might contribute to national health and welfare. This was in response to the criticism of the Bhore Committee report (1946) that it did not cede a place to Indigenous medicine in planning for health and medical care in independent India.[42]

This report (1948) makes fascinating reading because it explicitly ceded the epistemological distinctiveness of Indigenous medicine and instead asserted that:

> We wish to emphasise here that the Committee do not believe in the multiplicity of systems of medicine. Science is universal and medical sci-

> ence is no exception. The so-called 'Systems' merely represent different aspects of and approaches to medical science as practised during different ages and in different parts of the world. Anything of value emerging from these should be utilised for the benefit of humanity as a whole without any reservation and integrated in the form of a unified system for the country.[43]

This is remarkable because in eschewing a distinct epistemic and cultural site for Indigenous medicine, this commission tried to assimilate Indigenous medicine and 'Western' medicine, which was configured as biomedicine and was in its supposedly golden age.[44] The members of the Commission were distinguished scholars and practitioners of Ayurveda and Tibbia; these included the principals of the Ayurvedic colleges in Banaras Hindu University and Madras University, the chair of the Board of Indian Medicine of the Bombay state, the principals of the Tibbia Colleges in Dhaka and Lahore, and the president of the Ayurvedic and Tibbia Board in Delhi. The two experts in Western medicine at the commission added at a later stage were the superintendent of Irwin Hospital in Delhi and the professor of pharmacology at the Carmichael Medical College in Calcutta. The Commission included representatives from the 'orthodox' schools of independent Ayurveda and Hakimi practitioners as well.[45]

Previous committees that examined the state of Indigenous medicine (and there had been several in colonial India) had focussed on four principal issues: the registration of legitimate practitioners to qualifications that would be recognised by the government; the pedagogy and funding for the institutionalisation of Indigenous medicine; the legitimacy and/or control of Indigenous drugs; and foremost, the use of the Indigenous medical practitioners to deliver medical care in rural areas. The political mobilisation of bodies of vaids and hakims intensified after provincial governments in Bengal, Bombay, Madras, Upper Provinces, and Punjab enacted legislation to prevent the government from employing unlicensed practitioners.[46]

Throughout the provincial legislatures of India when they acquired the portfolio of health after 1919, the governments of Bengal, Upper Provinces, Madras, Berar and C.P., Bombay, and Assam commissioned ways of delivering basic medical facilities through the training and appointment of Indigenous medical practitioners. Their recommendations differed a little in details but each provincial committee in colonial India agreed on several points: that Indigenous medicine was used by a large majority of Indians; that the therapies available were of a widely varying standard; that the practitioners likewise differed greatly in expertise and skills; and that medical care everywhere except in urban areas lacked (qualified) Western medical practitioners and Indigenous medical practitioners could be trained to practise medicine at these sites. Some provinces, for instance, the Upper Provinces, opted for a limited employment of Indigenous medical practitioners in government curative institutions at subordinate levels.[47] Even before the provincialization of the health portfolio, the Bombay government allowed for the municipal funding of an Ayurvedic dispensary in Poona after popular mobilisation in its favour.[48] The Bombay government allowed local bodies to finance Ayurvedic dispensaries in some areas and commissioned a report in 1947 that went much further. It recommended sustained research in Ayurvedic drugs and laid down a framework for the modernization of pedagogy in Indigenous medicine through government support.[49] In Madras province, the government allowed the registration of Indigenous medical practitioners in 1933, and a decade before, on the recommendations of the Usman committee, the government established a college for the training of Ayurveda and Unani practitioners in Madras.[50] The Madras college offered a four-year training program in Indigenous medicine, which was to be supplemented by one year of study in Western medicine techniques including surgery. The Punjab government report, published in 1941, echoed similar sentiments and cited the Madras government's strategy as the model for the future of Indigenous medicine in the province.[51] By 1949, the Assam government had allocated funds for a board of Indian medicine for the establishment of an Ayurvedic college in Guwahati.[52] Almost all provincial governments in late colonial India, therefore, concurred on the usefulness of Indigenous medical practitioners *if* they were skilled in Western medical knowledge, had knowledge of Ayurvedic or Unani medical systems, and knowledge of Indigenous drugs. To this end, most states in independent India established boards of Indian medicine and colleges with extended curricula, including training in anatomy, physiology, and biomedicine. The all-India committee of 1948 endorsed the establishment of colleges and a restructured curriculum to 'integrate' Indigenous and Western medicine: "The Committee are convinced that an integration of the Ayurvedic, the Unani and the Western is both possible and practicable."[53] The report placed the burden of integration largely on practitioners of Indigenous medicine and dismissed suggestions that the attempt at 'synthesis' might result in the Indigenous medical systems being 'swallowed up':

> The Committee have come to the conclusion that there should be no … apprehension on the part of Vaidyas and Hakims if they have any real faith in the strength of the Science and the Art of the medicine they practice. Through investigation and research into their fundamental theories they should be able to show that their medicine is equally strong, scientific and based on solid foundation … If they cannot do this, their systems have no right to exist. They should, therefore boldly face the prospect of integration and synthesis … and agree to the pooling of all that is best anywhere to alleviate suffering and to combat disease.[54]

The postcolonial nation-state continued to support the institutionalisation of Indigenous medicine through a government ministry and the establishment of Indigenous medical colleges. As Anthony Cerulli pointed out through textual and anthropological research, the integrated curriculum enabled graduates of Indigenous medical colleges to be employed in biomedical clinics, dispensaries, and hospitals in subordinate positions 'through the back door' in contemporary India.[55] Scholars have interpreted this trajectory as 'modernisation' or 'globalisation' of Indigenous medicine, and so it is. However, this adaptation into the medical culture of consumption globally by manufacturers of Ayurvedic medicines self-consciously inhabits the space of providing alternative therapies to biomedicine. There is no pretension of epistemic synthesis or equivalent status. When borrowings take place, these are of personnel whose skills are adapted and move only in one direction – from Indigenous medical therapies to biomedical treatments.[56] The objectives of self-sufficiency in drugs for the new nation-state, therefore, were not fulfilled by intensive research in Indigenous drugs; historical momentum was with the invention of new synthetic drugs and the expansion of the biomedical-industrial complex. The contributions of Indigenous medicines were relegated to the realm of the alternative.

Conclusion

Medical Cultures in Modern India

I began this book with thoughts on the contemporary pharmaceutical industry in India and its transformation after the TRIPS agreement in 2005. A fundamental turn that made the manufacture of generic drugs possible on a large scale through the Patent Act of 1970 was abandoned by India's agreement with the World Trade Organization (WTO) and Trade Related Aspects of Intellectual Property Rights (TRIPS). This was part of a process of structural transformations in the Indian economy as well as in world trade that began in the 1990s.[1] Simultaneously, transnational firms' interest in Indigenous drugs assumed political interest and critical urgency in intellectual property rights through the now infamous case of the American firm that tried to patent the derivatives of the common neem tree.[2] Meanwhile, Ranbaxy, one of the largest pharmaceutical firms in India that manufactured generic life-saving drugs like anti-retrovirals and exported these to developing countries, was found to have systematically violated Food and Drug Administration (FDA) norms of quality in manufacture and supply.[3] The scholarly consensus among social scientists that refers to the Act of 1970 as the moment that Indian pharmaceutical firms could decolonize the industry ignores the multiple strands and prior histories of the industry.[4] As several chapters in this book have shown, the urgent and topical themes of production of cheap generic medicines, selective appropriation (bio-prospection/bio-piracy) of Indigenous drugs, the pervasiveness of substandard and fake drugs, the lack of qualified pharmacists and doctors or the access to them by the poor, and practices of self-medication with hundreds of licit and illicit drugs belong to longer narratives from the nineteenth century.

Medicines and their dissemination, quality, prices, and potency as well as the identities of their dispensers and debates about these in the public sphere were fundamental aspects of India's colonial modernity. Therefore, dreams of a distinct pharmacopeia, the validation of Indigenous drugs, or self-sufficiency in medicines for the nascent nation were raised and found great resonance in colonial India.The nationalist aspirations for legitimisation of Indigenous drugs and achievement of self-sufficiency in drugs production engendered medical discourse among doctors as well as vaids and hakims, was debated in both the nationalist and the loyalist presses and informed government policy at the centre and in the provinces. The principal fissure in medical discourse was not between Western medical practitioners and vaids and hakims, although these 'encounters' did highlight the state's bias towards Western medical institutions and medicines imported from Britain. Instead, the fundamental divergence in colonial India was between those who were prepared to accept Indigenous drugs within Western pharmacopeia after their active principles were identified and others who used the Indigenous drugs from the local markets. The latter comprised the largest proportion of medical practitioners in colonial India. Medical praxis and the medical market itself were eclectic and dynamic.

This book has argued that this eclectic approach was replicated at the stage of production and in the contexts of dissemination of medicines and other therapeutic commodities. Many reformers among vaids and hakims took to producing drugs on an industrial scale, encased them in modern packaging, and marketed them through advertisements in print and on billboards and flyers. At the same time, the local drug manufacturing industry involved older occupational castes as well as newly educated scientific professionals who produced therapeutic commodities based on Indigenous drugs and the BP. This thriving medical market was supported by industrialization within princely states like Baroda and Mysore. The colonial government was the largest manufacturer, importer, and consumer (through the army and civil hospitals) in British India, and it limited its remit to supplying medicines to a handful of institutions that met the needs of the government. Government policy on the quality or standardization of drugs or of training of medical professionals was light and implemented only loosely; instead, the ire of official and medical discourse rested largely on the racialized 'bazaar medicines' and their purveyors, the bazaar pharmacists as well as the notoriously non-standardized Indigenous drugs. The consumers, producers, and distributors of modern medicines in colonial India were as disparate as the remedies in the market.

Medical Pluralism and the Global South

Historians have explained the transformations in the cultures of medicine in modern India through its articulations in the public sphere, in nationalist politics, and in caste and community assertions of identity that created new communities of practitioners and consumers.[5] These studies have remained distinct from any historical examination of drugs or their manufacture or dissemination. The latter appears to pose a separate set of queries on colonialism and drug regimes, international diplomacy and maritime trade, or new recreational cultures of narcotic drugs.[6] Therefore, historical reflections on the production and distribution of drugs and their reception and consumption have remained separate and distinct. Contemporary writings on the circulation of spurious drugs in India, meanwhile, abstain from historical reflection.[7] Anthropologists have more fruitfully raised queries about the production of drugs as well as their circulation in the global South. These have emphasised how pharmaceuticals are formulated or acquire distinct cultural and economic meanings in specific, localized contexts and have usefully examined medicalization as well as pharmaceutalisation in a globalized world.[8] Although culturally distinct, one common theme to have emerged from these and similar studies is the ubiquity of plural medical cultures *and* the simultaneous expansion of biomedicine in poorer countries.

The diverse and heterogeneous medical market in colonial India was entrenched through historical processes that involved imperial tariffs, piecemeal colonial legislation, nationalist assertions both cultural and economic, and a vastly unequal colonial society. This book has demonstrated that the medical market emerged and expanded in colonial India through distinctive colonial policies. These included limited manufacture and distribution of medicines by government agencies for a restricted number of establishments and an unregulated market for the rest. The plurality in this market can be seen at different sites – at the eclectically educated compounder who gave himself the title of 'Dr' and dispensed medical advice to pharmacists who marketed diluted or outdated medicines to consumers with lighter pockets. Therefore, medical pluralism in contemporary India is not only the consequence of globalization in the twenty-first century.

Medical Cultures in Modern India

This book has tried to emphasise that medical cultures in modern India have not been just diverse and heterogeneous but also ideologically flexible and materially adaptable. This is less a celebratory sentiment than an observation of the structural inequities entrenched in colonial as well as postcolonial society in India. A few who have access to these use high-quality drugs and take recourse to curative institutions that offer medical care from qualified professionals. The vast majority cannot afford the high costs of quality drugs, and they are served by the grey market – medicines of lesser potency and medical practitioners of dubious qualification. In 1931, when the DEC sent questionnaires to the diverse community of doctors, vaids and hakims, pharmacists, and reputed manufacturers of therapeutic commodities, there was near unanimity on the need for stricter drug control legislation, although their views on the means to do so differed. A few medical men, practising privately or even in government employ, pointed out that stricter drug laws would raise the prices of drugs still higher, making these unaffordable to most Indians.[9] Although it took several years, drugs legislation and drugs standardization laboratories were in place in 1945.[10] Yet, proprietary drugs of dubious merits and diluted or outdated medications continued to serve the market, as did large numbers of compounders and doctors of uncertain qualification and training. The Pharmaceutical Committee (Bhatia) report of 1954 reiterated that:

> The Committee … feels convinced that … the drugs in the Indian market are not above reproach and that many of them are of impure quality and defective strength. The evidence points to … the traffic in such

> drugs is extensive and indiscriminate … adulteration, deterioration or tampering with the quality or strength of drugs, very little distinction can be made between imported and locally manufactured medicinal preparations.[11]

I have argued for a nuanced interpretation of 'adulteration' in chapter 5. This is not to legitimize fraudulent and exploitative practices at the expense of the-poverty-stricken citizenry who received unacceptably inefficacious medicines. I would highlight, instead, that the drug control regime, significant though it was, did not impede the brisk trade in non-standardized medical therapies. In the 1950s, in the wake of the therapeutic revolution and with patents on sulphonamides and antibiotics, transnational pharmaceutical firms became prominent in the USA. With concerns about the cheapness and safety of the new drugs under vast monopolies of pharmaceutical firms, a US senate sub-committee chaired by Ester Kefaveur investigated the drug industry's patents and monopolies.[12] As the Kefaveur committee in the USA found out, the price of drugs in India was one of the highest in the world in the 1950s, much of it owing to the monopolistic practices of transnational firms that continued to trade in India.[13] In the Nehruvian era, the government manufacturing plants of antibiotics and synthetic drugs were established to facilitate easier access to cheaper and efficacious drugs.[14] Their manufacturers did not keep pace with the overall demand and transnational firms continued to dominate the medical market. When the Ayyangar Committee (1959) reported that inventions could be classified as 'non-patentable' if they intervened with the national economy or 'national health or well-being', the right to health was seen as being in conflict with monopolistic patent rights and this eventually paved the way for the Patent Act of India (1970).[15] This allowed only process and not product patents, thereby generating a slew of Indian pharmaceutical firms that manufactured generic life-saving drugs and marginalized transnational firms in India. Therefore, the Patent Act of India is celebrated as the catalyst for the flourishing generic drug industry in India.

And yet, the incremental government regulations, postcolonial planned manufactures, and even the expansion of the private sector in the pharmaceutical markets have not eliminated or substantially eroded the disparate and eclectic cultures of medical praxis in modern India. Scholars may argue that this is the consequence of the hyper commodification and 'reformulation' of the Indigenous, especially Ayurvedic, drug industry, particularly in the postcolonial era.[16] It appears commonsensical that this pluralism is intrinsic to any society that has limited and hierarchical access to biomedical treatments and institutional care. After all, it is not only in India but in much of the global South that the entry of biomedicine and medical consumerism elicited competition with local curative praxis. As historians have noted, integrative medicine achieved state support in China in the mid-twentieth century. There was a thick seam of Hindu sectarian (as well as Hindu nationalist) rhetoric in much of the plea for state support for Indigenous medicine in colonial India that referenced ancient (and pre-Islamic) knowledge. However, as vaids appropriated minor technologies like injection syringes and stethoscopes in daily diagnostic practice, reformists among vaids and hakims also called for restructuring their pedagogy to include the study of anatomy, general pathology, and chemistry.[17] When the Committee for Indigenous Medicine submitted its report in 1948, it firmly pointed in the direction of integrating Indigenous medicine with scientific medicine:

> We believe that, while Indian medicine can take much of practical value from the Western medicine, the latter can also learn much from the philosophic background of Indian system, its comprehensiveness, the importance it attaches to the soil factor and dietary, its generalisation of principles and the knowledge of truth gained by the use of supra-sensory perception.
>
> … Opinion in favour of integration .leading to synthesis has been expressed by exponents of Western end Indian medicine and by the prominent members of the lay public and we are of opinion that immediate steps should be taken in this direction.[18]

Streamlined syllabi and official degrees in Indigenous medicines and separate medical colleges for these were supported by the Indian state. Nonetheless, state policy remained heavily in favour of biomedicine and infrastructure based on biomedical solutions. Therefore, by the 1950s, any vision of integrative medicine faded away. However, its informal and unaccountable counterpart, medical pluralism, is embedded in everyday lives in all parts of the global

South. Notwithstanding grim predictions, the pharmaceutical industry in India has changed its priorities and adjusted to the post-TRIPS regimen to the extent of remaining a lucrative and growing sector. Meanwhile, access to medicines remains uncertain or expensive for most.

Notes

Introduction

1 See Bell and Figert, 'Medicalization and Pharmaceuticalization', 775–83. The scholarly literature on pharmaceuticalisation has focussed on consumer-oriented medicalisation in the postcolonial global South. I have borrowed the term for use with reference to colonial and postcolonial society in India because the consumer culture in pharmaceutical/therapeutic commodities in India pre-dated the independent nation-state.

2 Monnais, *The Colonial Life of Pharmaceuticals*; Mukharji, *Doctoring Traditions*; Banerjee, 'Ayurveda in Modern India', 201–14.

3 Greene, *The emergence of India's Pharmaceutical Industry*, 1–41; Agarwal et al., *A Failure of Regulatory Diligence*; see also, Thakur, 'Ranbaxy Was Never the Exception', 59; Winstanley, 'This World: Bad Medicine', 165.

4 Chaudhuri, 'Multinationals and Monopolies, 46–54.

5 Wadman, 'Falsified Data'.

6 Shukla and Sangal, 'Generic Drug Industry in India', 236–40.

7 Al Dahdah, Kumar, and Quet, 'Empty Stocks and Loose Paper', 778–95; Saha and Hossain, 'Evaluation of Medicines Dispensing Pattern', 1–8.

8 Haynes, *Rhetoric and Ritual in Colonial India*. For a discussion of public space and identity in colonial princely India, see Nair, 'Modernity and "publicness"', 5–29.

9 Freitag, *Collective Action and Community*; Dalmia, *The Nationalization of Hindu Traditions*; Arunima, 'Imagining Communities–Differently', 63–76.

10 Orsini, *The Hindi Public Sphere.*

11 Chatterjee, *The Nation and Its Fragments.*

12 Perkins, 'From the Mehfil to the Printed Word', 47–76.

13 Naregal, *Language Politics, Elites, and the Public Sphere.*

14 Mantena, 'Vernacular Publics and Political Modernity, 1678–1705.

15 Appadurai, 'Public Modernity in India', 1–20.

16 The scholarship on this theme is rich. See Rai, 'Invoking "Hindu" Ayurveda', 411–26; Mukharji, *Doctoring Traditions*; Berger, *Ayurveda Made Modern*; Sharma, *Indigenous and Western Medicine*; Hardiman, 'Indian Medical Indigeneity', 263–83; Ganesan, 'Medicine and Modernity', 108–31; Islam, 'Indigenous Medicine as Commodity', 777–98; Sivaramakrishnan, *Old Potions New Bottles*; Banerjee, 'Power, Culture and Medicine', 435–67; Panikkar, 'Indigenous Medicine and Cultural Hegemony', 283–308; Leslie, 'The Ambiguities of Medical Revivalism', 356–67.

17 Attewell, *Refiguring Unani Tibb*; Alavi, *Islam and Healing.*

18 Quaiser, 'Politics, Culture and Colonialism', 317–55; Quaiser, 'Science, Institution and Colonialism', 523–61.

19 Hardiman and Mukharji, 'Introduction'.

20 Ibid.

21 As Burton Cleetus has shown, the Ezhavas, an 'untouchable' healing caste in Kerala, negotiated with both the colonial state and Ayurveda practitioners; by streamlining their medical practises to satisfy the 'rationality' of scientific medicine and the high tradition of Ayurveda, they acquired a higher social status for themselves as well as their medicine. Cleetus, 'Subaltern Medicine and Social Mobility', 147–72.

22 Gupta, 'Procreation and Pleasure', 17–44.

23 There are several excellent recent studies of subaltern medical cultures and their dynamic characteristics. See, for instance, Barrett, *Aghor Medicine*; Lambert, 'Medical Pluralism and Medical Marginality', 1029–36; Blaikie, 'Mainstreaming Marginality', 145–72.

24 Mukharji, *Nationalizing the Body.*

25 Das, *Vernacular Medicine in Colonial India.*

26 Baer, 'Divergence and Convergence', 176–93; Warner, 'Physiological Theory and Therapeutic Explanation', 235–57; Basford, 'A Historical Perspective', 1261–9; Winter, 'Ethereal Epidemic', 1–27; Marland and Adams, 'Hydropathy at Home', 499.

27 Mukharji, *Doctoring Traditions.*

28 Berger, *Ayurveda Made Modern*; Other scholars have identified these trends as

well. See, for instance, Rai, 'Invoking "Hindu" Ayurveda', 411–26. Nor was this process of 'purifying' religious practice from syncretising healing traditions limited to Hindus; once the Sikhs consolidated their communal identity in British India, Sikh leaders similarly disseminated literature that forbade worship at heterodox or syncretic healing shrines. See Oberoi, 'The Worship of Pir Sakhi Sarvar', 29–55.

29 Cerulli, 'Politicking Ayurvedic Education'.

30 Arnold, *Colonizing the Body*.

31 Mishra, *Pilgrimage, Politics, and Pestilence*.

32 Chandavarkar, 'Plague Panic and Epidemic Politics', 203–40.

33 Roger, *The Politics of Health in India*. For a recent argument that colonial public health was confined to specific and privileged sites, see Bhattacharya, *Contagion and Enclaves*.

34 Harrison, *Public Health in British India*.

35 Ramanna, *Western Medicine and Public Health*.

36 Arnold, 'Medical Priorities and Practice', 167–83; Harrison, *Public Health in British India*; Ramasubban, 'Public Health in British India', 38–60.

37 There is rich literature on the army and cultures of sexual policing in India. See Ballhatchet, *Race, Sex, and Class*; Kaminsky, 'Morality Legislation and British Troops', 78; Levine, 'Venereal Disease, Prostitution, and Politics', 579–602; Chatterjee, 'The Indian Prostitute', 51–5; Levine, 'Rereading the 1890s', 585–612; Peers, 'Soldiers, Surgeons and the Campaigns', 137–60; Legg, 'Stimulation, segregation and Scandal', 1459–505.

38 Chakrabarti, 'Medicine amidst War and Commerce', 1; Harrison, *Public Health in British India*.

39 Arnold, 'Cholera and Colonialism in British India', 118–51.

40 Watts, 'From Rapid Change to Stasis', 321–74; Watts, 'Cholera and the Maritime Environment', 19–38; Isaacs, 'DD Cunningham and the Aetiology of Cholera', 279–305; Harrison, 'A Question of Locality', 133–59.

41 For a graphic narrative of how infants were used to transport live Jennerian vaccines, see Arnold, *Colonizing the Body*. See also, Arnold, 'Touching the Body', *The British Empire: Critical Readings Principles* 3 (2019); Catanach, '"The Gendered Terrain of Disaster"', 241–67.

42 Harrison, introduction to *From Western Medicine to Global Medicine*.

43 Arnold, *Colonizing the Body*, 57; Bhattacharya, 'The Genesis of Hospital Medicine', 231–64.

44 Colonial policies reified the caste system. The tension between keeping the caste

hierarchy stable and reinforcing a modern and Christian discourse of freedom from caste remained an enduring aspect of colonialism throughout.

45 Chakrabarti, *Materials and Medicine*, 53, 89.

46 After Partha Chatterjee's *Nation and Its Fragments,* it has been impossible to look at the gender question in colonial India without referring to the private/public spheres of nationalist discourse where women were metaphorically placed within the cloistered and domestic space.

47 Lal, 'The Politics of Gender and Medicine', 29–66; Lang, 'Drop the Demon Dai', 357–78.

48 Hardiman, *Missionaries and their Medicine.*

49 British medical officials tended to categorize knowledge of Indigenous drugs on the part of Ayurveds and Hakims as 'empirical', by which they meant that they knew what ailments the drugs could be used for but did not have scientific knowledge of their properties or of their active ingredients. See, for instance, 'Indigenous Drugs', *Indian Medical Gazette*, September 1879, 260–2; 'The Field for Research in Indian Indigenous Drugs', *Indian Medical Gazette,* December 1922, 467–9.

50 Warner, *The Therapeutic Perspective*, 5–6. See also, Rosenberg, 'The Therapeutic Revolution', 485–506.

51 Arnold, *Colonizing the Body*; Bhattacharya, 'The Genesis of Hospital Medicine', 231–64.

52 Sehrawat, *Colonial Medical Care.*

53 Harrison, *Public Health in British India.*

54 The 'pice-packets', comprised powders of quinine or its alkaloids in doses of 5 grams each, were produced at government-owned quinine factories and were intended for prophylactic use for large sections of the population in districts where malaria was endemic. See Barton, '"The Great Quinine Fraud"', 6–25.

55 Sivaramakrishnan, *Old Potions New Bottles*; Berger, *Ayurveda Made Modern*; Quaiser, 'Science, Institution and Colonialism', 523–61; Metcalf, 'Nationalist Muslims in British India', 1–28.

56 Wallis, 'Exotic drugs and English Medicine', 20–46; Cook and Walker, 'Circulation of Medicine', 337–51.

57 Simmons, 'Stills, Status, Stocks and Science', 141–61; German firms challenged the British dominance in global drugs in the mid-nineteenth century, enabled mostly through advanced research in chemistry and industrialisation. Cramer, 'Building the "World's Pharmacy"', 43–73. For a comparison of the drugs market through

industrialisation and transformation through the chemical revolution between Germany, Britain, and the USA, see Liebenau, 'Ethical Business', 116–29.

58 Harrison, *Medicine in an Age of Commerce and Empire.*

59 Chakrabarti, *Materials and Medicine.* This form of appropriation from the non-Western botanical world, once it was rationalised into long-term industrial production of pharmaceuticals in the late nineteenth century, is identified as bioprospecting. For an analysis of bioprospection of botanical drugs from Africa for transnational pharmaceutical firms, see Osseo-Asare, *Bitter Roots.*

60 Attewell, 'Interweaving Substance Trajectories', 1–20; Mukharji, 'Vishalyakarani as Eupatorium Ayapana', 65–87; Winterbottom, 'Of the China Root', 22–44.

61 Anderson, 'Travelers, Patent Medicines, and Pharmacopeias', 63–82. For an example of how a 'foreign' therapeutic product was assimilated widely within Indian society, see Mills, 'Drugs, Consumption, and Supply', 345–62.

62 I have repeatedly referred to Ayurvedic/Unani-Tibb as these were the dominant medical systems. But these systems were heterogeneous and accommodated multiple variants, and there prevailed in colonial India other lesser-known medical systems and innumerable therapies. The Indian subcontinent was not an exception here, most colonial nations accommodated plural medical systems and numerous remedies. See, for instance, Au, *Mixed Medicines*; Monnais, *The Colonial Life of Pharmaceuticals.*

63 Edwards, 'Bitter Pills', 21–58; Deb Roy, *Malarial Subjects*; Yang, 'Selling an Imperial Dream', 101–25.

64 As Michael Worboys has shown, medical research into malnutrition and vitamins led to a depoliticisation of food in medical and scientific discourse and a tendency to favour technical solutions, i.e., vitamin pills rather than identify the structural problems of hunger. See Worboys, 'The Discovery of Colonial Malnutrition'. In colonial India, however, the medical research on malnutrition was focussed mostly on beri-beri and little affected government intervention. See Arnold, 'British India and the "Beriberi Problem"', 295–314.

65 Historians of modern Chinese medicine have more easily identified how Chinese medicine integrated multiple influences, including Western medical therapies and praxis, changing the character of what is presently known as Traditional Chinse Medicine (TCM). See Andrews, *The Making of Modern Chinese Medicine.* Moreover, the state in China, both nationalist and then the communist regimes, actively participated in enhancing and sustaining the reformed Chinese medical system. See Lei, *Neither Donkey nor Horse.*

Chapter One

1 Gandhi's 'anti-modernity' or radicalism, expressed most clearly in *Hind Swaraj*, represents the clearest facet of the rejection of Western institutions. Bilgrami, 'Thinking Radically with Gandhi', 3–16; Chatterjee, *Nationalist Thought and Colonial India*, 86–130.

2 Arnold, *Everyday Technology*, 3–13.

3 Chaudhuri, 'Modernity at Home', 221–40.

4 Gerth, 'Consumption and Nationalism'.

5 Arnold, 'Global Goods and Local Usages', 407–29; Haynes, 'Masculinity, Advertising and the Reproduction', 23–46; Misra, *The Indian Middle Classes*.

6 Sharma, 'Creating a Consumer'.

7 S. Prasad has demonstrated that this self-conscious discourse of the middle classes in colonial Calcutta evoked a supposedly lost rural ideal where their items of daily consumption – milk, fish, mustard oil – had supposedly been uncontaminated. The inference is that the commercially available items of consumption in the cities were impure and imperfect, still it is at these sites that they were marketed and consumed. Prasad, 'Crisis, Identity, and Social Distinction', 245–65; Chatterjee, '"New Wine in New Bottles"', 94–108.

8 Johnson, 'Commodity Culture', 70–4; See also, Ombongi, 'The Historical Interface', 353–72; Anderson, *Pharmacy and Professionalization*, 99–128; Pearn, '"Where There is No Doctor"', 162–80; Hendriksen, 'Consumer Culture, Self-Prescription, and Status', 147–67.

9 Stepan, *Picturing Tropical Nature*.

10 Arnold, *The Tropics and the Traveling Gaze*.

11 Wallis, 'Exotic Drugs and English Medicine', 20–46; Wallis, 'Consumption, Retailing, and Medicine', 26–53.

12 Drayton, *Nature's government*; Brockway, 'Science and Colonial Expansion', 449–65.

13 Roberts, 'The Politics of Professionalization', 37–56; Holloway, 'Producing Experts, Constructing Expertise', 116–40.

14 Church, 'The British Market for Medicine', 281–98.

15 Johnson, 'Commodity Culture', 70–4.

16 Dorner, *Merchants of Medicines*.

17 Joshi, ed., *The Middle Class in Colonial India*.

18 Anderson, 'The Drugging of the Empire'.

19 Extract from the Proceedings of Indian Legislative Council, Proceedings July 1916, Nos 38–50 GOI/Home/Medical A, NAI/Delhi, 47.

20 For a discussion on the private medical schools that burgeoned in Calcutta, see Arnold, *Colonizing the Body*, 1–11; Harrison, *Public Health in British India*.

21 S.K. Sawday, Officiating District Collector of Jalpaiguri to Commissioner of Rajshahi, 4 Aug 1913, Government of Bengal/Finance/Med, November 1913, 119–20.

22 Quaiser, 'Politics, Culture and Colonialism', 317–55.

23 Tansey, 'Medicines and Men', 411–16.

24 *Bruce and Co's Companion to the Tropical Medicine Chest in which are Described the Virtues and Doses of Medicines, with a Popular View of the Symptoms and Treatment of Tropical Diseases and other useful information, Drawn up for the Guidance of the Indian Sojourner; with special reference in regard to Professional Aid*. (Madras: Vepery Mission Press 1843, v.

25 *Bruce and Co's*, xi.

26 White, *Companion to the Medicine Chest*, vi.

27 Kerr, *The A.B.C. of Domestic Medicine*.

28 Thompson, *Handy book of Directions*, i.

29 WF/M/GB/01/12/02, Ff 89. See also WF/M/GB/01/12/02, Ff91, WF/M/GB/01/12/02, Ff96, WF/M/GB/01/12/02, Ff105. Wellome Collections, London.

30 Chakrabarti, 'Medical Marketplaces Beyond the West', 196–215; Harrison, 'From Bazaar Medicine to Hospital Medicine', 61–79.

31 Government Central Branch Press, Shimla, *Annual Administration Report of Medical Store Department*, 1909–1910, 1910, 1.

32 'Medical Supplies to Local and Municipal Boards', *Indian Medical Record*, 1 March 1894, 148.

33 The prosperous princely state of Baroda in western India, for instance, regularly used both the pharmaceutical manufacturing and trading firms of Treacher and Co. and Kemp and Co of Bombay to order the delivery of medicines, chemicals for photography, telescopes, opera glasses, cigars, and wines and spirits. See Baroda Record Office, Huzoor English Office, Merchants and Tradesmen, 99/127/19, 1875–79.

34 Hervey, *The European in India*, 33.

35 Renford, *The Non-Official British in India*.

36 To give just one example, George Allen, a British adventurer who went to India around 1850, initially traded in tooth powder and hair oil. He went on to own the influential Anglo-Indian newspaper published from Allahabad, *The Pioneer* and

joined with partners to establish Cooper, Allen and Company, a large manufacturing firm that supplied boots to the Indian Army; Yalland, *Boxwallahs*, 220–1.

37 'A Report of the Exhibits of Drugs, Chemicals, Instruments, etc. in the Calcutta International Exhibition', *The Chemist and Druggist*, 15 March 1884, 115.

38 John A. Falck, 'Pharmacy in India', *The Chemist and Druggist*, 9 April 1887, 441–2.

39 Ramamurthy, *Imperial Persuaders*, 24–62; Burke, *Lifebuoy Men, Lux Women.*

40 'Editorial: A Valuable Trade', *Indian and Eastern Druggist*, January 1922, 19–20.

41 Hogg, *Practical Remedies*, iii.

42 *Guide to Poona and Kirkee, with directory, for the season 1876, etc.*, compiled by Treacher and Co, Ltd, Chemists, Wine and General Merchants, Bombay, Byculla, and Poona, 1876.

43 Keene, *Handbook for Visitors*, 27.

44 *Directory of Cawnpore*, 1907.

45 Hervey, *The European in India*, 65.

46 Allen, 'Pharmacy at a Hill Resort in India', 733.

47 'Pharmacy in India', *The Chemist and Druggist*, 16 Febrary 1889, 239.

48 For instance, see *Bombay Guardian*, 5 January 1901, 1.

49 GOI//Foreign Department Internal B. Feb. no 258/59, Dec 11, 1906 NAI (Delhi), 7.

50 'A Report of the Exhibits of Drugs, Chemicals, Instruments, etc. in the Calcutta International Exhibition', *The Chemist and Druggist*, 15 March 1884, 115.

51 Ibid.

52 Letter from Burroughs to Henry Wellcome, 25 July 1883, 5, Wellcome Collections.

53 Furedy, *British Tradesmen and Shopkeepers of Calcutta*, 9; Also see, Compton, *Indian Life*, 145.

54 Fellows Medical and Manufacturing Co. to B.W. & Co., Bombay 19 May 1882, Wellcome Collections, London.

55 Ibid.

56 For instance, the firm of Gillian and Company, who traded at Lahore, were the first British-owned firm to establish their medical store at Simla. WF/E/02/01/01/06, February 1997, Wellcome Collections, London.

57 Compton, *Indian Life*, 141.

58 'The Dak Bungler', *The Pioneer Mail and Indian Weekly*, 16 April 1890, 519.

59 'East Indian News', *The Chemist and Druggist,* 20 August 1904, 357.

60 *The Chemist and Druggist*, 7 February 1920, 80–1; *Indian and Eastern Druggist*, April 1920, 15.

61 Anderson, *Pharmacy and Professionalization.*

62 *Alphabetical List of Drugs, Medicines and Other Preparations Free from, and Containing, Spirit, compiled from the Results in Tests Made by The Customs Houses at Calcutta, Bombay, and Madras*, Madras, Superintendent, Govt Press, 1903, 1.
63 Church and Tansey, *Burroughs, Wellcome & Co.*.
64 Burroughs to C.W. White, *Canvassing India Thoroughly*, 1883, 5, Wellcome Collections, London.
65 Henry Wellcome to Mr T.H.B. Long, March 11, 1903, 254, Wellcome Collections, London.
66 See chapter 6 'From Compounder to Pharmacist' for methods of dispensing medicines and medical advice.
67 'Tabloid Hypodermics', Monthly Memo Points for Propaganda, May 1932, 328, Wellcome Collections, London.

Chapter Two

1 P.C. Ray in particular is identified as the pioneering chemist-industrialist in colonial India. Recent scholarship has continued with nationalist frameworks of understanding P.C. Ray and the history of the B.C.P.W. See Basu, *History of Indigenous Pharmaceutical Companies*; Sarkar, 'In Pursuit of Laxmi', 459–514; Sen, 'Imperial Policy and Travails of Indigenous Enterprise'.
2 For a more nuanced approach that nonetheless locates the trajectories of the BCPW and the Alembic Chemical Works as nationalist enterprises stifled by lack of technological innovation as well as capital and protectionist tariffs see Chakrabarti, 'Science and Swadeshi', 117–42; Tripathi, '"Colonial Syndrome"', 121–41; Tyabji, *Colonialism, Chemical Technology and Industry*.
3 'Current News on Export Trade: India and Ceylon', *Chemist and Druggist* 66 (1905): 375.
4 B.W. and Co. to W.E. Smith, 28 March 1906, Wellcome Collections, London.
5 John A. Falck, 'Pharmacy in India', *The Chemist and Druggist*, 9 April 1887, 441–2.
6 'The Chemist and Druggist Trade in Calcutta', *Indian Medical Record* 3 (1 September 1892): 350.
7 Such complaints spanned some fifty years until the Drugs Enquiry Committee of 1931. See, for instance, 'Pharmacy in India', *Chemist and Druggist* 33 (1888): 552; 'Indian Incursions', *The British and Colonial Druggist* (31 March 1911): 257; 'Indian Drugs Inquiry', *Chemist & Druggist* 114, no. 27, 249.
8 'India and the German Traders', *The Indian Trade Journal* (April 1908): 100–1.

9 Station Press, Simla, *Report of the Committee of the Punjab Trades Association, 1st April 1916 to 31st March 1917*, 1918, 10–11.

10 Bently, 'The "Extraordinary Multiplicity" of Intellectual Property Laws', 161–200.

11 Home/Public Proceedings 362–5, NAI (New Delhi) August 1889, 1–2.

12 Home/Public Proceedings 362–5, NAI (New Delhi) August 1889, 1–2.

13 Chopra, 'Drug Adulteration and Spurious Drugs in India', 693.

14 'The History of a Pharmacy', *Indian Medical Record* 29 (1909): 185.

15 *Chemist and Druggist* 104 (1926): 757–60.

16 *Chemist and Druggist* 93 (1921): 70.

17 O'Meara, *Medical Guide for India*, 647–8.

18 'Bombay Medical Congress: From the pharmaceutical point of view', *The Pharmaceutical Journal and Pharmacist* (20 March 1909), 409.

19 *Chemist and Druggist* 96 (1922): 45.

20 *Indian and Eastern Druggist* 2 (1921): 194.

21 'Local purchase of certain articles for X-ray department', IOR/ P/11321, (APAC), Bombay Medical, 1923, 373.

22 *All India Swadeshi Directory* (Ahmedabad: Gujarat Sahitya Mandir 1931), 385–8.

23 Commerce/June 1922, IOR/P/11247, 3–59. Asian and African Collections, British Library London.

24 Commerce/June 1922, IOR/P/11247, 109. Asian and African Collections, British Library London.

25 For a fuller account of the Swadeshi movement in its earlier phase, see Sarkar, *Swadeshi Movement in Bengal.* The Indian National Congress organized the first Indian Industrial and Agricultural Exhibition in 1901, in Calcutta. The next was in 1902, in the industrial city of Ahmedabad, and then the exhibition moved successfully to Bombay, Madras, and Benares; all intensely urban, manufacturing, or trading centres. By the time it came around again to Calcutta in 1906–07, it attracted manufacturers from all over India, covered an area of 22 acres and included about a thousand exhibitors. Industrial India Office, Calcutta, 1907, *A Report of the Indian Industrial and Agricultural Exhibition, Calcutta, 1906-7*, v.

26 Industrial India Office, Calcutta, 1907, *A Report of the Indian Industrial and Agricultural Exhibition, Calcutta, 1906-7*, xxii.

27 Industrial India Office, Calcutta, 1907, *A Report of the Indian Industrial and Agricultural Exhibition, Calcutta, 1906-7*, 106–13.

28 See, for instance, Chakrabarti, 'Science and Swadeshi', 117–42; Tripathi and Mehta, *Business Houses in Western India*, 116–30.

29 Ray, 'Bengal Chemical and Pharmaceutical Works', 91.
30 Ray, 'Gospel of Charkha, Lament of a Spinner', 361–78.
31 Ray, *Life and Experiences*, 92–3.
32 Ibid., 97–100.
33 Ibid., 101.
34 Ibid., 103.
35 Ibid.
36 Ibid., 104.
37 Mehta, 'Institution Building in Princely India', 669–77.
38 Shah, *Baroda by Decades*, 104.
39 Raina and Habib, 'Technical Institutes in Colonial India', 2619–24; Mehta, 'Institution Building in Princely India'.
40 Nanavati, *Notes on Industrial Development*, 14–15.
41 Singh, 'Tribhovandas Kalyandas Gajjar', 419–29.
42 Amin, *The Rise and Growth*, 2–5.
43 Tyabji, *Colonialism, Chemical Technology and Industry*.
44 Bhagavan, 'Demystifying the "Ideal Progressive', 385–409.
45 Hardiman, 'From Custom to Crime', 165–228; See also, Hardiman, 'Purifying the Nation', 41–65.
46 Hardiman, 'From Custom to Crime', 165–228.
47 Memo 96 of 1907–1908, General Daftar 200/61, Huzur Political, Baroda Record Office.
48 From 1911, the ACWL was to export alcohol to Bombay State from Baroda. General Daftar 200/70 A, Huzur English Office, Revenue (Abkari) 1911-19, Baroda Record Office, 27–32.
49 Baroda Economic Development Committee 1918-19, Bombay, *The Times Press*, 1920, 146–7.
50 Excise Commissioner's office Baroda to Government of Bombay, 12 Oct 1915, Huzur English, General Daftar 200/70 A. Baroda Record Office, 35–9.
51 Chadwick, 'Industrial Development in India', 656–8.
52 See the correspondence between the Dewan of Baroda's office and the Government of Bombay, General Daftar 240, File 110 (IMFL) Huzur Political, Baroda Record Office between 1917–1919, especially Manubhai N Mehta, Dewan (prime minister) Baroda state to Baroda Resident's Office, Dec 9, 1918, 23–9.
53 ACWL to GOI, Finance Dept, Central Board of Revenue, Customs Duties, 6 April 1938, File no 706-Cus.I/38. Year- 1938. NAI, 1–5.

54 See correspondence between NCWL, Navsari, and Baroda Durbar and with the B.B. & Central Railways, 1934–8. Huzur Political/Revenue/Abkari200/244/169, Baroda Record Office.

55 See correspondence between NCWL, Navsari, and Baroda Durbar and with the B.B. & Central Railways, 1934–8. Huzur Political/Revenue/Abkari200/244/169, Baroda Record Office, 33–6.

56 Nair, *Mysore Modern*; Sen, 'The Beginning of Biochemical Researches', 37–50; Basu, 'Chemical Research in India', 591–600.

57 Kumar, Joshi, and Ram, 'Sandalwood', 1408–16.

58 *Chemist and Druggist*, 30 July 1921.

59 Baldwin, *Industrial Growth in South India.*

60 Mysore Pharmaceuticals, Bangalore to GOI Simla, 11 March 1925, NAI/Govt of India/Central Board of Revenue/Excise and Opium 195 E.O. 25, 1925, 1–3.

61 Ibid.

62 Attewell, 'Compromised', 369–86.

63 'Looking Ahead', *Indian Drugs and Pharmaceuticals* 1, no. 1 (May-June 1966): 15.

64 Roy, 'The Origins of Import', 71–95.

65 Sharma, *Indigenous and Western Medicine*; Haynes, 'Selling Masculinity', 787–831.

66 Mukharji, *Nationalizing the Body*, 179–211.

67 Leslie, 'Pluralism and Integration', 401–17.

68 Zandu Pharmaceutical Works Limited, Bombay, *Suchipatra: Dar ni Avritti [Index and List of Prices]*, Bombay, 1937, 1.

69 *Suchipatra: Dar ni Avritti*, 2.

70 Ibid., 3.

71 Ibid., 14.

72 Ibid, 15.

73 Ibid, 59.

74 Drugs Enquiry Committee Report 1931, 63.

75 Inamdar, *Rokda*.

76 Quaiser, 'Science, Institution, Colonialism', 523–62; Attewell, *Refiguring Unani Tibb*; Metcalf, 'Nationalist Muslims in British India', 1–28.

77 Bode, 'Taking Traditional Knowledge', 225–36.

78 Banerjee, 'Power, Culture and Medicine', 435–67.

Chapter Three

1 Indian Pharmacopoeia Committee, *Pharmacopoeia of India*. This was the first pharmacopeia of India.

2 There were several such compendiums in English, compiled by and officially endorsed for use by government medical officials. The first of these was W.B. O'Shaughnessey's *Bengal Dispensatory*. See O'Shaughnessy, *The Bengal Dispensatory*. Prior to this, Whitelaw Ainslie's *Materia Medica* served to translate and inform medical officials of some of the common drugs in use in regional Indian markets. See Ainslie, *Materia Medica of Hindoostan*.

3 Cartwright, *The British pharmacopoeia*; Anderson, 'Pharmacopoeias of Great Britain', 1–8.

4 Winterbottom, 'Of the China Root', 22–44; Attewell, 'Interweaving Substance Trajectories'.

5 Waring, *Pharmacopœia of India*.

6 Waring, *Remarks on the Uses*.

7 General Medical Council, *Indian and Colonial Addendum to the British Pharmacopœia, 1898*, Government of India Edition, 1901 (London: Spottiswoode & Co., 1900).

8 da Costa, 'Geographical Expansion', 74–81.

9 Grove, 'Indigenous Knowledge', 121–43.

10 Wallis, 'Exotic Drugs and English Medicine', 20–46.

11 Grove, 'Indigenous knowledge', 121–43.

12 Even in 1870, an army surgeon's manual in British India contained instructions for ordering supplies of a number of bazaar drugs each month, including alum, camphor, 'country' sulphur, catechu, mustard and linseed oils, and pomegranate root. See Fraser, *The British Medical Officer's Indian Manual*, 73.

13 Chakrabarti, 'Medical Marketplaces', 196–215.

14 Hardiman, 'Indian Medical Indigeneity', 263–83. David Hardiman has pointed out that this rediscovery of Sanskrit medical texts was a fragmented and chaotic affair because many the texts were closely guarded by the families who had inherited them over generations; manuscripts that were accessible were often incomplete and almost always included later interpolations and additions.

15 Cohn, 'Law and the colonial state', 131–52; Michael R. Anderson, 'Islamic Law and the Colonial Encounter', 165–85; Mani, 'Contentious Traditions', 119–56.

16 Ainslie, *Materia Medica of Hindoostan.*

17 Panikkar, 'Indigenous Medicine and Cultural Hegemony', 283–308.

18 Hardiman, 'Indian Medical Indigeneity', 263–83; Sivaramakrishnan, *Old Potions, New Bottles*; Attewell, *Refiguring Unani Tibb*, 206–7; Berger, *Ayurveda Made Modern.*

19 Mukharji, *Nationalizing the Body*; Sharma, *Indigenous and Western Medicine*; Gupta, 'Procreation and Pleasure', 17–44.

20 Kumar, 'Unequal Contenders, Uneven Ground'; Alavi, *Islam and Healing.*

21 Mukharji, 'What's in a Name?', 3–25; See also, Mukharji, 'Pharmacology, "Indigenous Knowledge", Nationalism', 195–212.

22 Mukharji, *Doctoring Traditions*. See also, Sharma, *Indigenous and Western Medicine*; Haynes, 'Creating the Consumer?', 185–223.

23 See, for instance, Batabyal, *A Manual of Unipathy*; Rao, 'A Plea for the Study of Indigenous Medicine', 187–94.

24 Mukharji, 'Pharmacology, "Indigenous Knowledge", Nationalism', 195–212.

25 Berger, 'Ayurveda and the Making', 101–16.

26 Waring, 'Preface to the Third Edition', in *Remarks on the Uses*, v–vii.

27 Calcutta Office of Superintendent, *Report of the Central Indigenous Drugs Committee of India* 1, Govt Printing, India, 1899. This committee was set up at the same time as a provincial Indigenous drugs committee instituted in the Madras Presidency.

28 'Indigenous Drugs of India', *Chemist and Druggist*, 1899, 536.

29 Dymock, Warden, and Hooper, *Pharmacographia Indica.*

30 Royle, *An Essay on the Antiquity of Hindoo Medicine.*

31 Ibid., vi.

32 Royle, *A Manual of Materia Medica and Therapeutics*, vii.

33 *The Pharmaceutical Journal and Transactions*, 1895, 651.

34 Dymock, Warden, and Hooper, *Pharmacographia Indica*, iii.

35 Ibid., 112–17.

36 Mukharji has made this argument in Mukharji, 'What's in a Name?', 3–25.

37 Basu, 'On the Study of Indigenous Drugs', 225–9, https://www.ncbi.nlm.nih.gov/pmc/issues/280155/#.

38 Kanny Lall Dey, 'Presidential Address, Section of Pharmacology', 25–8.

39 Editorial, 'The Use of Indigenous Drugs in India', *The Pharmaceutical Journal*, 30 November 1895, 464.

40 'Indigenous Drugs of India', *Chemist and Druggist*, 1 April 1899, 536.

41 'The Indian and Colonial Addendum to the British Pharmacopœia', *The Lancet* 157, no. 4039 (1901): 267–8.

42 'The Extra Pharmacopoeia', *Indian Medical Gazette* 36, no. 7 (July 1901): 272, https://www.ncbi.nlm.nih.gov/pmc/issues/281272/#.

43 'Service Notes', *Indian Medical Record* 36, no. 1 (Jan 1901): 40, https://www.ncbi.nlm.nih.gov/pmc/issues/281269/#.

44 Ibid.

45 For a discussion on the persistence of the idea of the tropical bodies being distinct and requiring distinctive treatment in the twentieth century, see Arnold, 'Diabetes in the Tropics', 245–61.

46 See, for instance, 'Eastern Systems of Medicine', *The Indian Review*, April 1916, 308; 'Investigation into Native Drugs', *Indian and Eastern Druggist*, July 1927, 149–50.

47 'Indian Pharmaceutical Industries', *Indian and Eastern Druggist*, December 1920, 15–16.

48 This point is discussed in detail in chapter 5.

49 Memo (Military no 142) from India Office, London (Salisbury) to the Governor General in Council, India, IOR/L/MIL/7/15141 [No 355, File 1] 8 June 1875 APAC, 5.

50 India Office, *Report of the Committee on the Supply of Drugs for India*, 1875, IOR/L/MIL/7/15141(APAC), 5–6.

51 GOI/Home/Medical A Proceedings (National Archives of India, New Delhi) July 1916, no. 38–50, 53.

52 Office of Superintendent, Calcutta, *Report of the Central Indigenous Drugs Committee of India, Vol. 1*, Government Printing, 1899, 60–3.

53 'Indian Drug Supplies', *The British and Colonial Druggist*, 28 April 1911, 942–3.

54 'Preface', *Medicinal Specialties* (BCPW Press, 1915), ii–iii.

55 Quirke and Gaudillière, 'The Era of Biomedicine', 441–52.

56 Chakrabarti, 'Empire and Alternatives', 75–94; Winterbottom, 'Of the China Root', 22–44.

57 P/11109, Government of Madras, Local/Municipal/ Public Health, (APAC), 1921.1.

58 V/27/850/41, Investigation of Indigenous Drugs, Government of Madras, Local and Municipal (Public Health) Department, 1921, (APAC), p.2.

59 Ayurvedas' associations in the Presidency complained bitterly and publicly about M.V. Koman's methods and expertise. See *Report of the Special Committee*

Appointed by the Joint Board of the Dravida Vaidya Mandal and the Madras Ayurveda Sabha in Reply to the Report on the Investigation into the Indigenous Drugs by Dr. M.C. Koman, Dravida Vaidya Mandal, *Vani Vilas Press, 1921.*

60 'Indigenous drugs', *Indian and Eastern Druggist*, September 1921, 217–18. See also, *Chemist and Druggist*, July 1921.

61 Chopra, *Indigenous Drugs of India*, 6.

62 Ibid., 39.

63 Government of India Central Publication Branch, *Report of the Drugs Enquiry Committee*, 1931, 136–46.

64 Government of India Central Publication Branch, *Report of the Drugs Enquiry Committee*, 1931, 144.

65 David and Vareed, 'Deterioration of the Digitalis Glucosides', 41–53.

66 'Indian Pharmacopeia', *Journal of South Indian Medicine* 3, no. 2 and 3 (15 February 1936): 47.

67 This is further discussed in chapter 7.

Chapter Four

1 Alter, 'Celibacy, Sexuality, and the Transformation of Gender', 45–66; Bhatia, 'Fashioning Women in Colonial India', 327–44; Nijhawan, 'Cumin, Capsules, and Colonialism', 170–97; Ray, 'The Body and its Purity', 395–421.

2 Leslie, 'The Ambiguities of Medical Revivalism', 356–67; Hardiman, 'Indian Medical Indigeneity', 263–83; Panikkar, 'Indigenous Medicine and Cultural Hegemony', 283–308; Attewell, *Refiguring Unani Tibb*.

3 Alavi, 'Unani Medicine', 101–29; Attewell, 'The End of the Line?', 387–419.

4 Quaiser, 'Politics, Culture and Colonialism', 317–55.

5 Mukharji, 'Baidya-as-Technology', 227–56; Berger, *Ayuveda Made Modern*, 36–7.

6 Bagchi, *Private Investment in India.*

7 Goswami, 'Sahibs, Babus, and Banias', 289–309.

8 Roy, *Traditional Industry.*

9 Haynes, 'Artisan Cloth-Producers', 170–98.

10 Arnold, 'Nehruvian Science and Postcolonial India', 360–70; Nayar, 'Nationalist Planning', 13–38; Chatterjee, 'Development Planning and the Indian State', 120–5.

11 See chapter 2.

12 Kumar, 'The Indian Drug Industry', 356–85.

13 See chapter 2.

14 Sehrawat, *Colonial Medical Care*; Harrison, *Public Health in British India*, 6–35.
15 Mazumdar, 'Reflecting on Chemical Education', 94–9.
16 'Sale of Medicines in Bengal', Home /Public, 1872, NAI, Oct. no 103, 1.
17 'Sale of Medicines in Bengal', Home /Public, 1872, NAI, Oct. no 103, 1. For an argument that quinine was used not just for malaria but more widely for a spectrum of symptoms and illnesses, see Deb Roy, *Malarial Subjects*.
18 APAC/IOR/L/MIL/7/15141 [No 355, File 1] Copy Military despatch to the GOI, no.191, July 20, 1876, 3.
19 APAC/IOR/L/MIL/7/15141 [No 355, File 1] Copy Military despatch to the GOI, no.191, July 20, 1876, 2.
20 APAC/IOR/L/MIL/7/15141 [No 355, File 1] Copy Military despatch to the GOI, no.191, July 20, 1876, 5.
21 For the transplantation and cultivation of cinchona in government plantations, see Mukherjee, 'Natural Science in Colonial Context'; Deb Roy, '"Fairest of Peruvian Maids"', in *Malarial Subjects*; For an overview of cinchona cultivation in British India, see Muraleedharan, 'Quinine (Cinchona) and the Incurable Malaria', 91–100; Nandini Bhattacharya, 'Contending Visions', in *Contagion and Enclaves*, 99–118.
22 APAC/IOR/L/MIL/7/15141 [No 355, File 1] Copy Military despatch to the GOI, no.191, July 20, 1876, 4.
23 Simmons, 'From Purgatives and Powders', 41–50.
24 Ibid. See also Anderson, 'The Drugging of the Empire', 19–22.
25 Simmons, 'From Purgatives and Powders', 41–50.
26 Apothecaries Hall, Blackfriars, London to Governor General-in-Council, India, 28 October 1875, APAC/IOR/L/MIL/7/15141 [No 355, File 1], 5.
27 Apothecaries Hall, Blackfriars, London to Governor General-in-Council, India, 28 October 1875, APAC/IOR/L/MIL/7/15141 [No 355, File 1], 5.
28 B.W. & Co., London to T.H.B. Long, 2 May 1902, Wellcome Collections.
29 APAC/IOR/L/MIL/7/15141 [No 355, File 1,].
30 'Pharmacy in the Indian Army by an old Qui Hai', *Chemist and Druggist*, 30 April 1904, 690–2.
31 Memo, Director of Public Instruction to DGIMS, 23 March 1900, General Department 1900, Maharashtra State Archive 65, 517.
32 Henry Wellcome to T.B.H. Long, 2 May 1902, Wellcome Letter Books, 908.
33 Government of India, List to Which Medical Supplies Will be Discontinued, etc., 2–4.

34 Government Of India, Contents of Part A of Proceedings of the Fin Dep (Mil Fin) May, no. 11–14, Medical, Orders 18 Sep 1906 and 1 May 1907.

35 Government Central Branch Press, Shimla, *Annual Administrative Report of Military Store Department, 1909–10*, 1910, 1.

36 Government Central Branch Press, Shimla, *Annual Administrative Report of Military Store Department, 1909–10*, 1910, 3.

37 Government Central Branch Press, Shimla, *Annual Administrative Report of Military Store Department, 1909–10*, 1910, 3.

38 Richards, 'The Opium Industry in British India', 149–80.

39 Government Central Branch Press, *Annual Report of Government Medical Store*, Simla, 1911, 9.

40 An Indian newspaper in Allahabad, *Indian People*, highlighted in 1909 the high prices charged by the Government Stores for quinine and claimed that this had led 'people to believe that the industry is being carried on for the sake of making money'. *Selections from the Native Newspapers Published in the United Provinces of Agra & Oudh.*, 1909. JSTOR, jstor.org/stable/saoa.crl.26082296. Accessed 13 Septempter 2021.

41 Government Central Branch Press, *Annual Report Government Medical Store, 1909–10*, Simla, 1910, 3.

42 Government Central Branch Press, *Annual Report Government Medical Store, 1909–10*, Simla, 1910, 3.

43 Government Central Branch Press, *Annual Report Government Medical Store, 1909–10*, Simla, 1910, 1–2.

44 Memo on the course of Military expenditure 1898–99 to 1912–13, Appendix 5, L/MIL/17/5/1903/APAC/BL, 72.

45 Memo on the course of Military expenditure 1898–99 to 1912–3, L/MIL/17/5/1903/APAC/BL, 17.

46 Chadwick, 'Industrial Development', 656–8; 'Industries after the War', *Journal of the Royal Society of Arts* 66, no. 3434 (1918): 669–72, http://www.jstor.org/stable/41347767.

47 *Report of the Indian Industrial Commission 1916–18*, Calcutta: Superintendent Government Printing Press, 1918, 56.

48 The Indian army's ordinance factories claimed to be the first industrial manufacturers in India but these too fell far short of urgent requirements for military guns/artillery and even ammunitions during the War. See H.A. Young, 'The Indian Ordnance Factories and Indian Industries', *Journal of the Royal Society of Arts* 72, no. 3715 (1924): 175–88, http://www.jstor.org/stable/41356452.

49 *Report of the Indian Industrial Commission 1916–18*, Calcutta: Superintendent Government Printing Press, 1918, 93–4.

50 For instance, see Tyabji, *Colonialism, Chemical Technology and Industry.*

51 Kumar, 'Reconstructing India', 241–57.

52 'India: Municipal Dispensaries', *Indian and Eastern Druggist*, December 1920, 9.

53 Roy, 'Equipping Leviathan', 398–423.

54 'The Mesopotamia Commission Report', *The Hospital*, 7 July 1917, 263–4; The shortages in supplies continued to affect the Indian army in the intermittent wars in the NWFP. See 'Headquarters' Failure in India', *The Hospital* 66, no. 1734 (August 1919): 531–2, PMID: 29832158.

55 For instance, the Smith, Stanistreet and Company exported the antiseptic Antipyrine (Phenazone) to London in July 1916, File no 82-83, Commerce & Industry (War) GOI/NAI, August 1916; Bathgate & Co. exported thymol to Glasgow in 1916, File no 49, Commerce & Industry (War) GOI/NAI, August 1916.

56 File no 20, April 1919 Customs (War)/Commerce &Industry/GOI/NAI, Delhi; File no 138-139, February 1919, Customs (War)/Commerce &Industry/GOI/NAI, Delhi; File no 217-218, February 1919, Customs (War)/Commerce &Industry/GOI/NAI, Delhi.

57 J.N. Dutt, 'Adulteration of Quinine', *Indian Medical Gazette* 51, no. 12 (December 1916): 474. PMID: 29008693; PMCID: PMC5315745.

58 Officiating Secretary, Government of Bengal, to Secretary to Government of India, June 20, 1919, NAI/GOI/Finance/Separate Revenue, B Proceedings, August 1919, no. 249–51, 5.

59 Dutt, *Commercial Drugs of India*, v–vi.

60 For instance, see 'Drug Cultivation in India', *Chemist and Druggist*, 25 October 1919, 81.

61 Even the government reported on the increased cost of medicines, although they were supplied by the GMS. For instance, see Bihar and Orissa (India), *Report on the Administration of the Territories Now Included in the Province of Bihar and Orissa*, 1914. *JSTOR*, jstor.org/stable/saoa.crl.26552615, accessed 26 August 2021.

62 In 1916, the *British Medical Journal* certified that the firm's preparation of thymol, a sample of it submitted to the *BMJ*, was of B.P. standard and capable of replacing thymol previously imported from Germany. See *British Medical Journal*, 22 April 1916, 593.

63 Rao, 'A Plea for the Study of Indigenous Medicine', 188–92.

64 Bode, *Taking Traditional Knowledge to the Market.*

65 'Tropical Climates and White Men', *Indian Medical Gazette* (November 1912):

497–9; 'Tropical Neuresthania', *Indian Medical Gazette* 63, no. 3 (March 1928): 150, https://www.ncbi.nlm.nih.gov/pmc/issues/284254/#; This was equally true of French colonies. See Monnais, *The Colonial Life of Pharmaceuticals.*

66 'The Future of Medicine in India', *Indian Medical Gazette* 56, no. 11 (November 1924): 563–7, https://www.ncbi.nlm.nih.gov/pmc/issues/281572/#.

67 Chopra, 'Some Aspects of Therapeutics in India', 151.

68 Sprawson, *Moore's Manual of Family Medicine*, 2–3.

69 Chatterjee, *Drugs of India.*

70 'New Patents', *The Pharmaceutical Journal and Pharmacist*, 11 December 1909, 744.

71 'On the Danger of the Use in India of So-Called Lactic Acid Bacilli Tablets Manufactured in Europe', *Food and Drugs* 1, no. 1 (July 1910): 15–22.

72 'The Indigenous Systems of Medicine', *Indian Medical Gazette* 57, no. 4 (1922): 141–2, https://www.ncbi.nlm.nih.gov/pmc/issues/282064/#.

73 Berger, *Ayuveda Made Modern*; Sivaramakrishnan, *Old Potions New Bottles.*

74 Attewell, *Refiguring Unani Tibb.*

75 Ghosh, 'The Scientific and Economic Importance of Research', 650–3.

76 DEC 1931, 221. (*Report of the Drugs Enquiry Committee, 1930–31.* Calcutta: Government of India Central Publication Branch, 1931.)

77 'Digitalis Preparations Sold in India', *The Indian Medical Gazette* 74, no. 7 (July 1939): 432–6, https://www.ncbi.nlm.nih.gov/pmc/issues/280810/#.

78 'The Drug and Pharmaceutical Industry in India', *The Indian Medical Gazette* 75, no. 9 (September 1940): 560–4, https://www.ncbi.nlm.nih.gov/pmc/issues/282202/#; See also, 'Indigenous Drugs Enquiry', *The Indian Medical Gazette* 75, no. 6 (June 1940): 367–70, https://www.ncbi.nlm.nih.gov/pmc/issues/282949/#.

79 McRobert, 'The Position of Medical Science in India', 607–11.

80 In 1875, quinine was expensive enough for medical officials to suggest that even the relatively privileged British troops in India who contracted non-malarious fevers be treated without using quinine through alternative methods of treatment, which 'would be productive of economy of a valuable and non-overabundant drug'. APAC/IOR/L/MIL/7/15141 [No 355, File 1] p.10.

81 'Conditions and Prospects of British Drug and Chemical Trades in India', *The Indian and Eastern Druggist*, April 1920, 15.

82 Government Central Press, *Report on the Proceedings of the Drugs Manufacture Committee, 1920*, Simla, 1920, 5–6.

83 The Jallianwalla Bagh massacre and its attendant horrors deeply influenced every strand of anti-colonial politics in India. For a survey of its political aftermath, see Ghosh, 'Whither India?', 389–97; Tuteja, 'Jallianwala Bagh', 25–61.

84 However, as the Indian Merchants' Chamber pointed out in 1922, even in the sectors where Indian industries were invited to submit tenders for government purchases, the Store Department continued to favour British manufacturers. See 'Chairman's Speech', *Annual Report of the Indian Merchants Chamber, 1923*, Bombay 1923, 32–6.

85 Government of India Central Publication Branch, *Report of the Drugs Enquiry Committee*, 1931, 131–5.

86 Government of India Central Publication Branch, *Report of the Drugs Enquiry Committee*, 1931, 245.

87 Government of India Central Publication Branch, *Report of the Drugs Enquiry Committee*, 1931, 408–9.

Chapter Five

1 See, for instance, Mishra, 'Food Adulteration, Public Health and Middle-Class Anxieties', in *Beastly Encounters of the Raj*, 102–20; Berger, 'Clarified Commodities', 1004–26.

2 Arnold, 'The "Discovery" of Malnutrition and Diet', 1–26.

3 Moore's manual and others; Arnold, 'Race, Place and Bodily Difference', 254–73.

4 There is rich scholarly literature on the politics of diet in colonial and post-colonial India. Gandhi, of course, highlighted diet as fundamental to the politics of nationalism. Food and drink or their renunciation remain embedded in political as well as social identities in modern India. See, for instance, Roy, 'Meat-Eating, Masculinity, and Renunciation', 62–9; Prasad, 'Crisis, Identity, and Social Distinction', 245–65; Michelutti, 'We are Kshatriyas but we Behave like Vaishyas', 76–95; Appadurai, 'How to Make a National Cuisine', 3–24.

5 Ray, 'The Body and its Purity', 395–421; Mukhopadhyay, 'Between Elite Hysteria and Subaltern Carnivalesque', 37–50.

6 T. Frederick Pearse, 'Beri Beri in Calcutta', *Indian Medical Record* 30 (April 1910): 45–6.

7 See, for instance, Burroughs Wellcome flyers in Tamil, Bengali, Hindi, and Gujarat warning against imitations Kepler Malt Extract and of Tabloid Cascara Sagrada. WF/M/GB/01/19/01Circular Book 18- 1912–13.

8 Arnold, *Toxic Histories*, 112.

9 Arnold, 'The Poison Panics', 49–71.

10 Evans and Bose, 'The Necessity for an Act Restricting'.

11 Arnold, 'The Poison Panics', 49–71.

12 *The Bombay Gazette*, 4 January 1895, 4.

13 The article was one of the public appeals from the scientific community that were influential in enabling the Government of India to enact the Indian Poisons Act of 1904. For an account of Chunilal Bose's public pronouncements on poisoning in the social life of Bengalis, see Arnold, 'Embracing Toxicity', in *Toxic Histories*.

14 *Chemist and Druggist*, 16 February 1889, 239.

15 Ibid.

16 'A Talk on the Indian Drug Trade', *Chemist and Druggist*, 19 July 1890.

17 'Proprietaries in India', *Chemist and Druggist*, 30 December 1899, 1077.

18 *Bombay Medical and Physical Society Proceedings* 9, no. 1 (20 January 1905): 5–61.

19 Ibid.

20 IOR/P/5645, GOI Medical, March 1899, APAC, British Library, 373–8.

21 See, for instance, the Appeal of Kanny Lal Dey in the first Indian Medical Congress in 1895, *The Pharmaceutical Journal and Transactions* 25, 1894–95, 446.

22 *The Chemist and Druggist*, 24 January 1903, 117.

23 Barton, 'Powders, Potion and Tablets', 142–61.

24 *The British and Colonial Druggist*, 26 August 1910, 183.

25 'Indian Drug Supplies', *The British and Colonial Druggist*, 12 May 1911, 381–2.

26 Sprawson, *Moore's Manual*, 1.

27 *Chemist and Druggist*, 4 March 1911, 38.

28 See chapter 3, note 51.

29 'Drugs for India', *The Chemist and Druggist*, 6 May 1911, 54.

30 Ibid.

31 'Drug Adulteration in India', *Indian Medical Gazette* (September 1911): 352–3, https://www.ncbi.nlm.nih.gov/pmc/issues/281522/#.

32 'Prevention of Adulteration', *The Indian Review* (April 1916): 307.

33 Khan, 'Food Adulteration in India'.

34 Prasad, *Cultural Politics of Hygiene*, 23–42.

35 Mishra, 'Food Adulteration'.

36 See also Ray, 'The Body and its Purity', 395–421; Sinha, *Colonial Masculinity*.

37 Arnold, 'An ancient race outworn', 123–43.

38 Ellis, 'If You Cannot Feed the Body of a Child'; Saha, 'Milk, Mothering & Meanings', 97–110.

39 See, for instance, Mishra, 'Food Adulteration'.

40 'Co-operation as Applied to Industrial, Particularly to Pharmaceutical Education', *Indian Medical Record*, April 1921, 79–80.

41 Chuckerbutty, 'The Present State of the Medical Profession in Bengal', 111.

42 Mukharji, *Nationalizing the Body.*

43 Das, *Vernacular Medicine in Colonial India.*

44 Andrews, *The Making of Modern Chinese Medicine*; Monnais, *The Colonial Life of Pharmaceuticals.*

45 See, for instance, 'Indigenous Drugs', *Indian Medical Gazette*, September 1879, 260–2, https://www.ncbi.nlm.nih.gov/pmc/issues/280639/#.

46 For Indigenous appropriation of homeopathy, see Das, *Vernacular Medicine in Colonial India.* For 'braiding' and appropriating western technology in Indian medical praxis, see Mukharji, *Doctoring Traditions.* For the symbiotic connects between Ayurvedic praxis and multiple forms of nationalism see Alter, 'Nature Cure and Ayurveda', 3–28; and Alter, *Gandhi's Body.*

47 'Adulteration of Drugs', *Indian Medical Record*, October 1925, 336.

48 National Archives of India, Commerce and Industry, Export of Quinine to Khartoum, Smith, Stanistreet & Co., May 1919, no. 98, P/9863; Revenue/Commerce and Industry, B Proceedings (June 1915), APAC, 137.

49 Supply of Defective Medical Stores by Messrs Phillips and Co. Bombay, 1916, APAC, IOR/L/MIL/7/15148/8.

50 'Medical News', *Indian Medical Gazette*, January 1939, 43–4, https://www.ncbi.nlm.nih.gov/pmc/issues/280804/#.

51 Pols, 'Notes from Batavia', 120–48; Harrison, '"The Tender Frame of Man"', 68–93; Kennedy, 'The Perils of the Midday Sun'; Livingstone, 'Tropical Climate and Moral Hygiene', 93–110.

52 N.B. Dutt, 'Some Thoughts on Indian Pharmacy', *Indian and Eastern Chemist* (December 1938): 376–8.

53 This argument was favoured by purveyors of Sino-Vietnamese medicines in colonial Vietnam as well. See Monnais, *The Colonial Life of Pharmaceuticals.*

54 Copy enclosure from S/G, 16th Nov 2876, NAI/GOI/MIL/ Despatch from Secretary of State 1877 Vol. 1. p.5.

55 Chowdhury, 'Medicine and Colonial Patent Law', 408–28.

56 As recent scholarship on medical advertisements in colonial India has demonstrated, these served local, small manufacturing firms that produced Indigenous as well as Western medicine as widely and successfully as it did the larger, transnational manufacturers. See, for instance, Sharma, *Indigenous and Western Medicine*, 120–35; Haynes, 'Selling Masculinity', 787–831; Haynes and McGowan, introduction to *Towards a History of Consumption in South Asia*, 1–25.

57 *Secret Remedies, What They Cost and What They Contain, Based on Analyses Made for the British Medical Association* (London, 1909).

58 Loeb, 'Doctors and Patent Medicines', 404–25; Bartrip, 'Secret Remedies, Medical Ethics', 191–204; See also, Digby, *Making a Medical Living*, 28.

59 Jenkinson, 'A "Crutch to Assist"', 1–36.

60 Haq, 'British Narco-diplomacy'.

61 For instance, the Indian Industrial Commission recommended that the government institute an Indian Chemical Service to provide chemical analysis for industrial processes in all industries. See Holland Committee Report, 1918, 236.

62 Kumar, 'Skilling and Its Histories', 249–71.

63 Block, 'European Drug Traffic and Traffickers', 315–37. For a study of how cocaine, which had to be imported into British India, became an item of casual consumption, see Mills, 'Drugs, Consumption, and Supply', 345–62.

64 Government of India Action on Drugs Enquiry Committee, File no 53-45/37-H 1937, Health Education and Lands/ Health, 8.

65 Government of India Action on Drugs Enquiry Committee, File no 53-45/37-H 1937, Health Education and Lands/ Health, 69.

66 Royal Society of Medicine Council to the Drugs Enquiry Committee, File no 53-45/37-H 1937, n.d. Health Education and Lands/ Health/NAI/New Delhi, 30.

67 T.S.S., et al., 'Science Notes A=and News', *Current Science* 8, no. 8 (1939): 388–95; R.N. Chopra and B. Mukerji, 'The Menace of Drug Adulteration in India', *The Calcutta Municipal Gazette: Eleventh Health Number*, 13 April 1940, 4–6 (South Asia Archive Online).

68 Manager of Publications, Delhi, *Report of the Health Survey and Development Committee*, 1946, 202–6.

69 *The Medical Bulletin*, 16 October 1937, 653.

70 'Drugs Bill', *Annual Report of the Indian Merchants Chamber, 1937* (Bombay: J.K. Mehta, 1938), 58.

71 Central Board of Revenue, Customs Duties, Govt of India, ACWL to GOI, Finance Dept, File no 706-Cus.I/38. Year- 1938, 6 April 1938, 7.

Chapter Six

1 Roberts, 'The Politics of Professionalization', 37–56; Crellin, 'Pharmaceutical History and its Sources', 215–27; Malleck, 'Professionalism and the Boundaries of Control', 175–98; Higby, 'Professionalism and the Nineteenth-Century American Pharmacist', 115–24.

2 Bennett, 'Passage through India', 201–20; Naraindas, 'Care, Welfare, and Treason', 67–96; Prashad, 'Marks of Capital', 1–30.

3 Kidambi, '"An Infection of Locality"', 249–67; Kamra, 'Law and Radical Rhetoric', 546–59.

4 Ryan and Khalid, *Public Health in the British Empire.*

5 Mukharji, *Doctoring Traditions.*

6 Ibid.

7 Eglash, introduction to *Appropriating Technology.*

8 Tilley, 'Global Histories, Vernacular Science', 110–19.

9 Alavi, *Islam and Healing.*

10 For a discussion on the emergence of private medical colleges and their graduates or students who failed to acquire the medical degrees but nonetheless practised as 'doctors', see Arnold, *Colonizing the Body.*

11 Sehrawat, 'Feminising Empire', 65–81; Pratik Chakrabarti, '"Signs of the Times"', 188–211; Jeffery, 'Recognizing India's Doctors', 301–26.

12 Harrison, *Public Health in British India.*

13 Jenkinson, 'A "Crutch to Assist"', 1–36.

14 John A. Falck, 'Pharmacy in India', *The Chemist and Druggist*, 9 April 1887, 441–2.

15 Ibid.

16 Ibid.

17 *Chemist and Druggist*, 26 August 1922, 309.

18 The most insightful scholarship on this theme is still Adas, *Machines as the Measure of Men.*

19 'Chemists' Assistants in India', *Chemist and Druggist*, 15 August 1908, 303–4.

20 *Chemist and Druggist*, 24 October 1908, 668.

21 'Illegal Use of Medical Titles', *Proceedings of Allahabad Medical Society* 1, no. 5 (October 1882): 120–2.

22 'East India News: Further Thefts by Compounders', *Chemist and Druggist*, 22 December 1900, 984.

23 Falck, 'Pharmacy in India', 441–2.

24 'Pharmacy in the Indian Army by an old Qui Hai', *Chemist and Druggist*, 30 April 1904, 690–2.

25 'Pharmacy in the Indian Army by an old Qui Hai', *Chemist and Druggist*, 30 April 1904, 690–2.

26 'Address by George Watt to the Pharmaceutical Society of Great Britain', *Chemist and Druggist*, 6 October 1906, 539–42.

27 Correspondence to Editor, 'Medical Registration for India', *The Medical Reporter*, 16 August 1894, 124.

28 Iswariah, 'The Pharmacy Bill', 334.

29 'Professional Monopoly', *Indian Medical Record* (22 March 1905): 8–10.

30 Reviews of *Sowlat Khan's Dispenser's Handbook*, *Indian Medical Gazette* 50, no. 12 (December 1915): 471, https://www.ncbi.nlm.nih.gov/pmc/issues/280769/#.

31 'Notes on Current Topics', *Indian Medical Gazette* 66, no. 12 (1931): 700–12, https://pubmed.ncbi.nlm.nih.gov/29010006.

32 'The Profession of Pharmacy', in *Drugs Enquiry Committee*, 1931, 73.

33 *Chemist and Druggist*, 22 April 1911, 36.

34 'Editorial: The Need for Reform', *Indian and Eastern Druggist*, June 1925.

35 *Report of Drugs Enquiry Committee*, 1931, 317.

36 Haynes, 'Selling Masculinity', 787–831.

37 Sharma, 'Creating a Medical Consumer'.

38 The proprietary medicine trade in India was robust from the late nineteenth century onwards, including American proprietaries as well as the more common and popular British and a few Continental ones. Anderson, 'Travelers, Patent Medicines, and Pharmacopoeias', 63–82.

39 'Proprietaries in India', 1077.

40 Anderson, 'Travelers, Patent Medicines, and Pharmacopoeias', 63–82.

41 The *Indian Trade Journal* 2, no. 21 (23 August 1926): 720.

42 'Conditions and Prospects of British Drug and Chemical Trades in India', *The Indian and Eastern Druggist*, April 1920, 15.

43 'Conditions and Prospects of British Drug and Chemical Trades in India', *The Indian and Eastern Druggist*, April 1920, 15. See also, *The Indian and Eastern Druggist*, July 1920, 25.

44 *Chemist and Druggist*, 19 May 1934, 579.

45 'Drugs and Medicines', *Chemist and Druggist*, 8 January 1938, 47.

46 *Chemist and Druggist*, 5 June 1926, 757–60.

47 Mair and Hull, *The European in India*, 303.

48 Mackintosh, 'The Legacy of the Patent Medicines Industry', 261–74.

49 Anderson, 'From "Bespoke" to "Off-the-peg"', 43–69.

50 Porter, *Health for Sale*.

51 Mackintosh, *The Patent Medicines Industry*; Tandon, 'Growth of Advertising Industry in India', 23622–5. In India, patent IMS officials noticed and wrote of

the use of the print medium for marketing patent medicines in the 1930s. See, for instance, Phipson, '"Patent" Medicines, the Public, and the Doctor', 98.

52 Haynes, 'Creating the Consumer?', 185–223; Sharma, 'Creating a Consumer', 213–28.

53 Chowdhury, 'Medicine and Colonial Patent Law', 408–28.

54 Selvanayagam, 'Pharmacy in Madras', 15–19.

55 Ibid.

56 Deposition by Mr W.J. Campbell, Smith & Campbell, Pharmaceutical Chemists, The Mall, Lahore, *Drugs Enquiry Committee, 1931*, 252.

57 Appendix B, Memoranda by Co-opted Members, *Report of the Drugs Enquiry Committee, 1931*, 208.

58 For instance, the Berry-White Medical School in Dibrugarh in Assam trained both 'licensed medical practitioners' and compounders who were subsequently employed at the British-owned tea estates in the region. See 'Medical, Research and Educational Institutions in India', *Seventh Congress of the Far Eastern Association of Tropical Medicine: Souvenir of the Indian Empire Being a Brief Description of the Chief Features of India and its Medical and Sanitary Problems*, Calcutta 1927, 260. See also, League of Nations Health Organisation Malaria Commission, *Report of the Malaria Commission on its Study Tour in India, Aug 23rd to Dec 28, 1929*, Geneva 1930, 51–2.

59 Capt. R.D. Willocks, District Medical and Sanitary Officer, Malabar, to Deputy Secretary Home/Med/GOI, 7 July 1911, no. 2121, P/10233/APAC/BL, 1–7.

60 Government of India Press, E.W.C. Bradfield, *An Indian Medical Review*, 1938, 250–2.

61 Bose, Mukerji, and Chopra, 'Quality of Quinine Preparations', 609.

62 Chopra and Mukerji, 'The Menace of Drug Adulteration', 1–5.

63 Selvanayagam, 'Pharmacy in Madras', 15–19.

64 Singh, 'India's Medico-Pharmaceutical Inheritance', 90–5; Kim, 'Adulterated Intermediaries', 939–77; Young, 'Patent Medicines', 648–56; For insight into American patent medicine industry, see Young, *The Toadstool Millionaires*.

65 Ministry of Commerce and Industry, Government of India Press, Report of the Pharmaceutical Enquiry Committee, 1954, 207.

66 Basak and Sathyanarayana, 'Pharmacy Education in India'; Basak and Sathyanarayana, 'Community Pharmacy Practice in India', 11.

Chapter Seven

1 Löfgren, ed., *The Politics of the Pharmaceutical Industry*; Chandran and Brahmachari, 'Policy as a Driver of Economic Growth', 1181–93.
2 Arnold, 'Nehruvian Science and Postcolonial India', 360–70.
3 Krishna, 'Organisation of Scientific Research'.
4 Quirke and Gaudillière, 'The Era of Biomedicine', 441–52; Lesch, *The First Miracle Drugs*.
5 Podolsky, *The Antibiotic Era*; Bud, *Penicillin: Triumph and Tragedy*.
6 Dale, 'Science in War and Peace', 280–3.
7 Rajadhyaksha, 'The Long Road', 43–60.
8 Kaviraj, 'Development Planning'; Kumar, 'Reconstructing India', 241–57; Arnold, 'Nehruvian Science and Postcolonial India', 360–70.
9 Bradfield, *An Indian Medical Review*.
10 Manager of Publications, Delhi, *Report of the Health Survey and Development Committee*, 1946.
11 For consensus on self-sufficiency and ideological contestations on the means of achieving this goal in postcolonial health care provisions, see Qadeer, 'Health planning in India', 51–75.
12 Harrison, *Medicine and Victory*, 182–231.
13 Mukherjee, *Hungry Bengal*.
14 'The War and the Supply of drugs', *The Pharmacist*, 1940, 3, 120–2.
15 Enclosure to the Private Secretary to the Viceroy's letter no 2886 dated 30/5/40 to the Private Secretary to the Secretary of State, IOR/L/E/8/1894, i-ii.
16 'Deputation to Indian Medical Director', *Chemist and Druggist* 137, Jan 1942, 69.
17 'War Production in India', *Chemist and Druggist*, 31 January 1942, 140.
18 Ibid.
19 Kemp and Company to Honorary Secretary, The Pharmaceutical and Allied Manufacturers' and Distributors' Association Limited, 28 November 1942, in 'Import and Supply of Medical Preparations', *Indian Medical Gazette* 78, no. 1 (Jan 1943): 62, https://pubmed.ncbi.nlm.nih.gov/29012287.
20 Chopra, 'Drug Manufacture in India', 233.
21 Tyabji, 'Negotiating Nonalignment', 37–60.
22 Review of *Haffkine Institute*, by S.S. Sokhey, *Current Science* 14, no. 10 (1945): 254–5, www.jstor.org/stable/24209410.

23 Sreenivasan, 'Pharmacy and Drug Legislation', 63–4; Chopra, 'The Drug Industry in India', 230.

24 Cutler et al., 'Mass Treatment of Syphilis', 377–439.

25 International Technical Assistance in Public Health, Penicillin Comes to South Asia, *Public Health Report* 67, no. 4 (1952): 333–57.

26 Chaudhuri and Chakravarti, 'Typhus in Calcutta', 43–51.

27 'Pharmacopaeias and Adjuvants', *Indian Medical Gazette* 89, no. 9 (1954): 539–41.

28 As emphasised, for instance, in the address of J.C. Ghosh to the Indian Pharmaceutical Association Congress in Calcutta on December 1950. See 'Research in Relation to the Development of the Pharmaceutical Industry', *Current Science* 19, no. 12 (December 1950): 373–4, http://www.jstor.org/stable/24212374.

29 Col. S.S. Sokhey, Report of Sub-Committee: National Health, National Planning Committee Series, Vora and Company, Publishers Ltd, Bombay, 1948, 50, https://ruralindiaonline.org/en/library/resource/national-planning-committee-series-report-of-the-sub-committee-national-health/.

30 Col. S.S. Sokhey, Report of Sub-Committee: National Health, National Planning Committee Series, Vora and Company, Publishers Ltd, Bombay, 1948, 50, https://ruralindiaonline.org/en/library/resource/national-planning-committee-series-report-of-the-sub-committee-national-health/.

31 Col. S.S. Sokhey, Report of Sub-Committee: National Health, National Planning Committee Series, Vora and Company, Publishers Ltd, Bombay, 1948, 214–16, https://ruralindiaonline.org/en/library/resource/national-planning-committee-series-report-of-the-sub-committee-national-health/.

32 J.C. Ghosh and R.C. Shah, Report of Sub-Committee: Chemical Industries, National Planning Committee Series, Vora and Company Publishers Ltd, Bombay, 1947, 117, http://hdl.handle.net/10973/45602.

33 'A Modern Drug Industry for India', *Current Science* 18, no. 2 (February 1949): 31–2, http://www.jstor.org/stable/24211880.

34 Tyabji, 'Negotiating Nonalignment', 37–60.

35 Tyabji, 'Gaining Technical Know-How', 331–49.

36 Tyabji, 'Gaining Technical Know-How'.

37 Government of India Press, *Report of the Pharmaceutical Enquiry Committee 1954*, 1954, 5.

38 Government of India Press, *Report of the Pharmaceutical Enquiry Committee 1954*, 1954, 68.

39 Confidential report on India April 1961, IOR/Mss Eur/158/265, 45.

40 K.M. Stedman, Assistant Secretary, to Scott McCarthy, Wellcome Building, London, 15 June 1961, IOR/Mss Eur/158/265, pp.1–2

41 Rao et al., 'India: Towards Universal Health Coverage', 587–98.

42 Ministry of Health, Government of India, *Report on the Committee on Indigenous Systems of Medicine, Vol. I*, 1948, 6–7.

43 Ministry of Health, Government of India, *Report on the Committee on Indigenous Systems of Medicine, Vol. I*, 1948, 8.

44 Historians have demonstrated how the 'therapeutic revolution' offered by antibiotics, although historically contingent, were proposed and marketed as cure-alls by pharmaceutical companies between 1960–80. See Greene, Condrau, and Siegel Watkins, eds, *Therapeutic Revolutions*. Antibiotics and their usage were debated in medical discourse from the start; but these related to the correct or 'rational' use, not to the clinical legitimacy of the antibiotics themselves. See Podolsky, *The Antibiotic Era*.

45 Ministry of Health, Government of India, *Report on the Committee on Indigenous Systems of Medicine, Vol. I*, 1948, 11–12.

46 Harrison, *Public Health in British India*, 35; *Mridula Ramanna*, 209; Muraleedharan, 'Professionalising Medical Practice', PE27–PE37; Sivaramakrishnan, *Old Potions New Bottles*.

47 Berger, *Ayurveda Made Modern*, 106–27.

48 Ramanna, 'Systems of Medicine', 3221–6.

49 *Report of the Indian Systems of Medicine Enquiry Committee, Bombay, 1947–48*, 29–36.

50 Muraleedharan, 'Professionalising Medical Practice', PE27-PE37; Wujastyk, 'The Evolution of Indian Government Policy'; Cerulli, 'Politicking Ayurvedic Education', 298–334.

51 Ministry of Health, Government of India, *Report on the Committee on Indigenous Systems of Medicine, Vol. I*, 1948, 49–53.

52 Ministry of Health, Government of India, *Report on the Committee on Indigenous Systems of Medicine, Vol. I*, 1948, 55.

53 Ministry of Health, Government of India, *Report on the Committee on Indigenous Systems of Medicine, Vol. I*, 1948, 82.

54 Ministry of Health, Government of India, *Report on the Committee on Indigenous Systems of Medicine, Vol. I*, 1948, 86.

55 Cerulli, 'Politicking Ayurvedic Education', 298–334.

56 Ibid.

Conclusion

1 Khanna and Singh, 'India's IPR Regime'.

2 Shiva, 'North South Conflicts', 501–8; Winterbottom, 'Becoming "Traditional"', 262–83.

3 Wadman, 'Falsified Data'; Brhlikova et al., 'Trust and the Regulation of Pharmaceuticals', 1–13.

4 Chaudhuri, *The WTO and India's Pharmaceuticals Industry.*

5 See, for instance, Das, *Vernacular Medicine in Colonial India*; Sharma, *Indigenous and Western Medicine*; Haynes, 'Selling Masculinity', 787–831; Mukharji, *Nationalizing the Body*; Sivaramakrishnan, *Old Potions, New Bottles*; Quaiser, 'Colonial Politics of Medicine', 29–42.

6 See, for instance, Deshpande, 'An Historical Overview of Opium Cultivation', 109–43; Legg, '"The Life of Individuals"', 647–64; Mills, 'Cocaine and the British Empire', 400–19.

7 Hodges, 'The Case of the "Spurious Drugs Kingpin"', 473–83.

8 For instance, see Geest and Reynolds Whyte, *The Context of Medicines in Developing Countries*; Reynolds Whyte, Geest, and Hardon, *Social Lives of Medicines*; Baxerres and Cassier, *Understanding Drugs Markets.*

9 For a few representative instances, see testimonies of Captain G. Srinivasamurthi, Messrs Madhava Menon, Murugesa Mudaliar, and Sankunni Menon (Representatives of the School of Indian Medicine, Madras), evidence from Lucknow by unnamed hakeems and proprietors of medical stores, and Dr K.S. Ray, Joint Secretary, Indian Medical Association Calcutta; *Appendices,* Drugs Enquiry Committee 1931, 9–10, 211–12, 263–5.

10 See chapter 5.

11 *Report of the Pharmaceutical Committee* (1954), 148; of Dr U. Rama Rao, co-opted member for Madras.

12 For a detailed note on the reasons for USA government's enquiry into antitrust monopolies in the 1950s, see Bud, 'Antibiotics, Big Business, and Consumers', 329–49.

13 For the relevance of the Kefauver committee's comments on drug prices in India, see Ghai, 'Patent Protection and Indian Pharmaceutical Industry', 43–8; for an overview of Estes Kesaveur anti-monopoly political campaign in USA, see Scroop, 'A faded Passion?'

14 See chapter 6.

15 Ayyangar, *Report on the Revision*, 21; Tulasi and Rao, 'A detailed study of patent system', 547.

16 Pordié and Gaudillière, 'The Reformulation Regime', 57–79.

17 Cerulli, 'Politicking Ayurvedic Education', 298–334; Mukharji, *Doctoring Traditions*; Berger, *Ayurveda Made Modern*.

18 Ministry Of Health, Government of India, *Report of the Committee on Indigenous Systems of Medicine, Vo1.* 1, 1948, 188.

Bibliography

Unpublished Records

British Library, London (Asia and Africa Collections)

India Office Records, Economic Department: Commerce and Revenue, 1921–24; Industries and Overseas, 1921–24; Economic and Overseas, 1924–46

India Office Records, Military Collections 1875–1915

India Office Records Government of Bombay Proceedings (Medical) 1913–28

India Office Records Government of Bengal Proceedings (Medical) 1890–1930

Private Papers: IOR/MSS/EU/F158/265 (Papers of the India, Pakistan and Burma Association (1941–72)

National Archives of India, New Delhi

Government of India Proceedings, Commerce and Industry

Government of India Proceedings, Education/Health

Government of India Proceedings, Finance/Central Board of Revenue/Customs

Government of India Proceedings, Finance/Central Board of Revenue/Excise and Opium

Government of India Proceedings, Foreign/Internal

Government of India Proceedings, Home/Medical

Baroda Record Room, Vadodara General Daftar (English)

Huzoor Political

Huzoor English Office

Wellcome Collections, Wellcome Library, London
Burroughs Wellcome and Company Letter Books
Silas Mainville Burroughs Papers/Business Correspondence
Wellcome Foundation/GB/Marketing/Circular Books

Periodicals

Antiseptic
The Bengalee
Bombay Guardian
The British and Colonial Druggist
British Medical Journal
Calcutta Medical Journal
The Chemist and Druggist
The Hospital
India Trade Journal
Indian and Eastern Druggist
Indian Drugs and Pharmaceuticals
Indian Medical Gazette
Indian Medical Record
Indian Medico-Chirurgical Review
Indian Punch
Journal of the Royal Society of Arts
The Lancet
Madras Medical Journal
The Medical Bulletin, A Fortnightly Journal for the Medical Practitioner
Medical Reporter
The Pharmaceutical Journal and Pharmacist
The Pioneer Mail and Indian Weekly
Proceedings of Indian Legislative Council
Proceedings of the Allahabad Medical Society
Proceedings of the Indian Merchants Chamber, Bombay
Swasthya (In Bengali)
Transactions of the Medical and Physical Society of Bombay

Official Reports

A Report of the Indian Industrial and Agricultural Exhibition, Calcutta, 1906–7. Calcutta: 'Industrial India' Office, 1907.

All India Swadeshi Directory. Ahmedabad: Gujarat Sahitya Mandir, 1931.

Alphabetical List of Drugs, Medicines and Other Preparations Free from, and Containing, Spirit, Compiled from the Results in Tests Made By The Customs Houses at Calcutta, Bombay, and Madras, 1. Madras: Superintendent, Govt Press, 1903.

Annual Administration Report of Medical Store Department, 1909–10. Simla: Government Central Branch Press, 1910.

Annual Administration Report of Medical Store Department, 1910–11. Simla: Government Central Branch Press, 1911.

Annual Administration Report of Medical Store Department, 1911–12. Simla: Government Central Branch Press, 1912.

Annual Administration Report of Medical Store Department, 1912–13. Simla: Government Central Branch Press, 1913.

Annual Administration Report of Medical Store Department, 1913–14. Simla: Government Central Branch Press, 1914.

Annual Administration Report of Medical Store Department, 1914–15. Simla: Government Central Branch Press, 1915.

Baroda Economic Development Committee 1918–19. Bombay: The Times Press, 1920.

Directory of Cawnpore, 1907.

Guide to Poona and Kirkee, with directory, for the season 1876, etc. Bombay, Byculla, and Poona: Treacher and Co, Ltd, Chemists, Wine and General Merchants, 1876.

Indian and Colonial Addendum to the British Pharmacopœia, 1898. Government of India edition, 1901

Report of the Committee of the Punjab Trades Association, 1st April 1916 to 31st March 1917.

Report of the Committee on Indigenous Systems of Medicine. Delhi: Ministry of Health, 1948.

Report of the Health Survey and Development Committee. Delhi: Manager of publications, 1946.

Report of the Pharmaceutical Enquiry Committee, Government of India. Delhi, Manager of Publications, 1954

Report of the special committee appointed by the Joint Board, the Dravida Valdya Mandal and the Madras Ayurveda Sabha, in reply to the report on the investigations into the indigenous drugs by M.C. Koman Avergal. Srirangam: Sri Vani Vilas Press, 1921.
Report of the Drugs Enquiry Committee, 1930–31. Calcutta: Government of India Central Publication Branch, 1931.

Published Books and Articles

Adas, Michael. *Machines as the Measure of Men: Science, Technology, and Ideologies of Western Dominance.* Ithaca: Cornell University Press, 1989.
Agarwal, Vinti, Omprakash K. Gupta, Karen Priyadarshini, and Shubham Agrawal. *A Failure of Regulatory Diligence: A Case Study of Ranbaxy Laboratories Ltd.* Fifteenth AIMS International Conference on Management, 2018.
Ainslie, Whitelaw. *Materia Medica of Hindoostan: And Artisan's and Agriculturist's Nomenclature.* Madras: Government Press, 1813.
Alavi, S. 'Unani Medicine in the Nineteenth-century Public Sphere: Urdu Texts and the Oudh Akhbar'. *The Indian Economic & Social History Review* 42, no. 1 (2005): 101–29.
Alavi, Seema. *Islam and Healing: Loss and Recovery of an Indo-Muslim Medical Tradition, 1600–1900.* Basingstoke: Palgrave Macmillan, 2008.
Alter, Joseph S. 'Celibacy, Sexuality, and the Transformation of Gender into Nationalism in North India'. *The Journal of Asian Studies* 53, no. 1 (1994): 45–66 https://doi.org/10.2307/2059526.
– *Gandhi's Body: Sex, Diet, and the Politics of Nationalism.* University of Pennsylvania Press, 2000.
– 'Nature Cure and Ayurveda: Nationalism, Viscerality and Bio-ecology in India'. *Body & Society* 21, no. 1 (2015): 3–28. https://doi.org/10.1177%2F1357034X14520757.
Amin, B.D. *The Rise and Growth of the Alembic Chemical Works: A History.* Baroda: Alembic Printing Press, 1939.
Anderson, Michael R. 'Islamic Law and the Colonial Encounter in British India'. In *Institutions and Ideologies: A SOAS South Asia Reader*, ed. David Arnold and Peter Robb, 165–185. Richmond, Surrey: Curzon Press, 1993.
Anderson, Stuart. 'The Drugging of the Empire: The Relationship between the Society of Apothecaries and the British East India Company 1706 to 1858'. *38th International Congress for the History of Pharmacy, Sevilla September 19–22, 2007.* 2007.
– 'From "Bespoke" to "Off-the-peg": Community Pharmacists and the Retailing of Medicines in Great Britain 1900 to 1970'. *Pharmacy in History* 50, no. 2 (2008): 43–69. http://www.jstor.org/stable/41112388.

– *Pharmacy and Professionalization in the British Empire, 1780–1970*. Basingstoke: Palgrave Macmillan, 2021.

– 'Travelers, Patent Medicines, and Pharmacopeias: American Pharmacy and British India, 1857 to 1931'. *Pharmacy in History* 58, no. 3–4 (2016): 63–82. https://doi.org/10.26506/pharmhist.58.3-4.0063.

Andrews, Bridie. *The Making of Modern Chinese Medicine.* Vancouver: University of British Columbia Press, 2014.

Appadurai, Arjun. 'How to Make a National Cuisine: Cookbooks in Contemporary India'. *Comparative Studies in Society and History* 30, no.1 (1988): 3–24. DOI:10.1017/S0010417500015024.

– 'Public Modernity in India'. In *Consuming Modernity: Public Culture in a South Asian World*, ed. Carol A. Breckenridge, 1–20. Minneapolis: University of Minnesota Press, 1995.

Arnold, David. '"An Ancient Race Outworn": Malaria and Race in Colonial India, 1860–1930'. In *Race, Science and Medicine 1700-1960*, ed. Waltraud Ernst and Bernard Harris, 123–43. London: Routledge, 1999.

– 'British India and the "beriberi problem", 1798–1942'. *Medical History* 54, no. 3 (2010): 295–314. https://doi.org/10.1017%2Fs0025727300004622.

– 'Cholera and Colonialism in British India'. *Past & Present* 113, no. 1 (1986): 118–51. https://doi.org/10.1093/past/113.1.118.

– *Colonizing the Body: State Medicine and Epidemic Disease in Nineteenth Century India*. Berkeley: University of California Press, 1993.

– 'Diabetes in the Tropics: Race, Place and Class in India, 1880–1965'. *Social History of Medicine* 22, no. 2 (2009): 245–61. https://doi.org/10.1093/shm/hkp005.

– 'The "Discovery" of Malnutrition and Diet in Colonial India'. *The Indian Economic & Social History Review* 31, no. 1 (1994): 1–26. https://doi.org/10.1177%2F001946469403100101.

– *Everyday Technology: Machines and the Making of India's Modernity*. Chicago and London: Chicago University Press, 2013.

– 'Global Goods and Local Usages: The Small World of the Indian Sewing Machine, 1875–1952'. *Journal of Global History* 6, no. 3 (2011): 407–29. http://dx.doi.org/10.1017/S1740022811000398.

– 'Medical Priorities and Practice in Nineteenth-Century British India'. *South Asia Research* 5, no. 2 (1985): 167–83. https://doi.org/10.1177%2F026272808500500208.

– 'Nehruvian Science and Postcolonial India'. *Isis* 104, no. 2 (2013): 360–70. https://doi.org/10.1086/670954.

– 'The Poison Panics of British India'. In *Anxieties, Fear and Panic in Colonial Settings: Empires on the Verge of a Nervous Breakdown*, ed. H. Fischer-Tiné, 49–71. Basingstoke: Palgrave Macmillan, 2016.

– 'Race, Place and Bodily Difference in Early Nineteenth century India'. *Historical Research* 77, no. 196 (200): 254–73. https://doi.org/10.1111/j.0950-3471.2004.00209.x.

– 'Touching the Body'. *The British Empire: Critical Readings Principles* 3 (2019).

– *Toxic Histories: Poison and Pollution in Modern India*. New York: Oxford University Press, 2016.

– *The Tropics and the Traveling Gaze: India, Landscape, and Science, 1800–1856*. Seattle: University of Washington Press, 2006.

Attewell, Guy. 'Compromised: Making Institutions and Indigenous Medicine in Mysore State, Circa 1908–1940'. *Culture, Medicine, and Psychiatry* 38, no. 3 (2014): 369–86. https://doi.org/10.1007/s11013-014-9390-y.

– 'The End of the Line? The Fracturing of Authoritative Tibbi Knowledge in Twentieth-Century India'. *Asian Medicine* 1, no. 2 (2005): 387–419. https://doi.org/10.1163/157342105777996548.

– 'Interweaving Substance Trajectories: *Tiryaq*, Circulation and Therapeutic Transformation in the Nineteenth Century'. In *Crossing Colonial Historiographies: Histories of Colonial and Indigenous Medicines in Transnational Perspective*, ed. Anne Digby, Ernst Waltraud, and Projit Mukharji. Cambridge: Cambridge Scholars Publishing, 2010.

– *Refiguring Unani Tibb: Plural Healing in Late Colonial India*. Hyderabad: Orient Longman, 2007.

Au, Sokhieng. *Mixed Medicines: Health and Culture in French Colonial Cambodia*. Chicago: University of Chicago Press, 2012.

Ayyangar, N. Rajagopala. *Report on the Revision of the Patents Law September, 1959*, SCC Online®, 2013.

Misra, Bankey Bihari. *The Indian Middle Classes: Their Growth in Modern Times*. Bombay: Oxford University Press, 1961.

Baer, Hans A. 'Divergence and Convergence in Two Systems of Manual Medicine: Osteopathy and Chiropractic in the United States'. *Medical Anthropology Quarterly* 1, no. 2 (1987): 176–93. DOI: 10.2307/648756.

Bagchi, Amiya Kumar. *Private Investment in India, 1900–1939*. Cambridge: Cambridge University Press, 1972.

Baldwin, George B. *Industrial Growth in South India: Case Studies in Economic Development*. Illinois: The Free Press, 1959.

Ballhatchet, Kenneth A. *Race, Sex, and Class under the Raj: Imperial Attitudes and Policies and Their Critics, 1793–1905*. London: Weidenfeld and Nicolson, 1980.

Banerjee, Madhulika. 'Power, Culture and Medicine: Ayurvedic Pharmaceuticals in the Modern Market'. *Contributions to Indian sociology* 36, no. 3 (2002): 435–67. https://doi.org/10.1177%2F006996670203600301.

Barrett, Ron. *Aghor Medicine: Pollution, Death, and Healing in Northern India*. Berkeley: University of California Press, 2008.

Barton, Patricia. '"The Great Quinine Fraud": Legality Issues in the "Non-Narcotic" Drug Trade in British India'. *The Social History of Alcohol and Drugs* 22, no. 1 (2007): 6–25.

– 'Powders, Potion and Tablets: The "Quinine Fraud" in British India, 1890–1939'. In *Drugs and Empires, Essays in Modern Imperialism and Intoxication, c. 1500–c.1930*, ed. James H. Mills and Patricia Barton, 142–61. Basingstoke: Palgrave Macmillan, 2007.

Bartrip, Peter. 'Secret Remedies, Medical Ethics, and the Finances of the British Medical Journal'. In *The Codification of Medical Morality*, 191–204. Dordrecht: Springer, 1995.

Basak, Subal Chandra, and Dondeti Sathyanarayana. 'Community Pharmacy Practice in India: Past, Present and Future'. *Southern Med Review* 2, no. 1 (2009): 11. https://pubmed.ncbi.nlm.nih.gov/23093872.

– 'Pharmacy Education in India'. *American Journal of Pharmaceutical Education* 74, no. 4 (2010): 68. https://doi.org/10.5688/aj740468.

Basford, Jeffrey R. 'A Historical Perspective of the Popular Use of Electric and Magnetic Therapy'. *Archives of Physical Medicine and Rehabilitation* 82, no. 9 (2001): 1261–9. https://doi.org/10.1053/apmr.2001.25905.

Basu, Aparajito. 'Chemical Research in India (1876–1918)'. *Annals of Science* 52, no. 6 (1995): 591–600. https://doi.org/10.1080/00033799500200421.

Basu, K.D. 'On the Study of Indigenous Drugs'. *Indian Medical Gazette* 27, no. 8 (August 1892): 225–9. https://www.ncbi.nlm.nih.gov/pmc/issues/280155/#.

Basu, Malika. *History of Indigenous Pharmaceutical Companies in Colonial Calcutta (1855–1947)*. London: Routledge, 2021.

Batabyal, B.B. *A Manual of Unipathy, or Sukshma-Ayurveda*. Batabyal, 1919.

Baxerres, Carine, and Cassier Maurice. *Understanding Drugs Markets: An Analysis of Medicines, Regulations and Pharmaceutical Systems in the Global South*. London: Routledge, 2021.

Bell, Susan E., and Anne E. Figert. 'Medicalization and Pharmaceuticalization at the Intersections: Looking Backward, Sideways and Forward'. *Social Science & Medicine* 75, no. 5 (2012): 775–83.

Bennett, Michael. 'Passage through India: Global Vaccination and British India, 1800–05'. *Journal of Imperial and Commonwealth History* 35, no. 2 (2007): 201–20. http://dx.doi.org/10.1080/03086530701337492.

Berger, Rachel. *Ayurveda Made Modern: Political Histories of Indigenous Medicine in North India, 1900–1955*. Basingstoke: Palgrave Macmillan, 2013.

– 'Clarified Commodities: Managing Ghee in Interwar India'. *Technology and culture* 60, no. 4 (2019): 1004–26. http://dx.doi.org/10.1353/tech.2019.0099.

Bhagavan, Manu. 'Demystifying the "Ideal Progressive": Resistance through Mimicked Modernity in Princely Baroda, 1900–1913'. *Modern Asian Studies* 35, no. 2 (2001): 385–409. http://dx.doi.org/10.1017/S0026749X01002049.

Bhatia, Nandi. 'Fashioning Women in Colonial India'. *Fashion Theory* 7, nos 3–4 (2003): 327–44. https://doi.org/10.2752/136270403778052050.

Bhattacharya, Jayanta. 'The Genesis of Hospital Medicine in India: The Calcutta Medical College (CMC) and the Emergence of a New Medical Epistemology'. *The Indian Economic & Social History Review* 51, no. 2 (2014): 231–64. https://doi.org/10.1177%2F0019464614525726.

Bhattacharya, Nandini. *Contagion and Enclaves: Tropical Medicine in Colonial India*. Liverpool: Liverpool University Press, 2012.

Bilgrami, Akeel. 'Thinking Radically with Gandhi'. *Social Scientist* 46, no. 11–12 (2018): 3–16. https://www.jstor.org/stable/26599994.

Blaikie, Calum. 'Mainstreaming Marginality: Traditional Medicine and Primary Healthcare in Himalayan India'. *Asian Medicine* 14, no. 1 (2019): 145–72. 10.1163/15734218-12341438.

Block, Alan A. 'European Drug Traffic and Traffickers between the Wars: The Policy of Suppression and Its Consequences'. *Journal of Social History* 23, no. 2 (1989): 315–37. http://www.jstor.org/stable/3787882.

Bose, Indu Bhusan, B. Mukerji, and R.N. Chopra. 'Quality of Quinine Preparations in Indian Hospitals and Dispensaries'. *The Indian Medical Gazette* 74, no. 10 (1939): 609. https://www.ncbi.nlm.nih.gov/pmc/issues/280820/#.

Bradfield, E.W.C. *An Indian Medical Review*. Delhi: Manager of Publications, 1938.

Brhlikova, Petra, Ian Harper, Nabin Rawal, Madhusudhan Subedi, and MR Santhosh. 'Trust and the Regulation of Pharmaceuticals: South Asia in a Globalised World'. *Globalization and Health* 7, no. 1 (2011): 1–13. https://doi.org/10.1186/1744-8603-7-10.

Brockway, Lucile H. 'Science and Colonial Expansion: The Role of the British Royal Botanic Gardens'. *American Ethnologist* 6, no. 3 (1979): 449–65. https://doi.org/10.1525/ae.1979.6.3.02a00030.

Bud, Robert. 'Antibiotics, Big Business, and Consumers: The Context of Government Investigations into the Postwar American Drug Industry'. *Technology and Culture* 46, no. 2 (2005): 329–49. https://doi.org/10.1353/tech.2005.0066.

– *Penicillin: Triumph and Tragedy*. Oxford: Oxford University Press, 2015.

Burke, Timothy. *Lifebuoy Men, Lux Women: Commodification, Consumption, and Cleanliness in Modern Zimbabwe*. Durham, North Carolina: Duke University Press, 1995.

Catanach, Ian J. '"The Gendered Terrain of Disaster"? India and the Plague, c. 1896–1918'. *South Asia: Journal of South Asian Studies* 30, no. 2 (2007): 241–67.

Cerulli, A. 'Politicking Ayurvedic Education'. *Asian Medicine* 13, no. 1–2 (2018): 298–334.

Chakrabarti, Pratik. 'Empire and Alternatives: Swietenia Febrifuga and the Cinchona Substitutes'. *Medical History* 54, no. 1 (2010): 75–94. doi:10.1017/S0025727300004324.

– *Materials and Medicine: Trade, Conquest and Therapeutics in the Eighteenth Century*. Manchester: Manchester University Press, 2010.

– 'Medical Marketplaces beyond the West: Bazaar Medicine, Trade and the English Establishment in Eighteenth-Century India'. In *Medicine and the Market in England and its Colonies, c. 1450–c. 1850*. London: Palgrave Macmillan, 2007.

– '"Neither of meate nor drinke, but what the Doctor alloweth": Medicine Amidst War and Commerce in Eighteenth-Century Madras'. *Bulletin of the History of Medicine* 80, no. 1 (2006): 1. https://doi.org/10.1353/bhm.2006.0009.

– 'Science and Swadeshi: The Establishment and Growth of the Bengal Chemical and Pharmaceutical Works, 1893–1947'. In *Science and Modern India: An Institutional History, c. 1784–1947*, ed. Uma Das Gupta, 117–42. New Delhi: Pearson Education, 2010.

– '"Signs of the Times": Medicine and Nationhood in British India'. *Osiris* 24, no. 1 (2009): 188–211. https://doi.org/10.1086/605975.

Chandavarkar, Rajnarayan. 'Plague Panic and Epidemic Politics in India, 1896–1914'. In *Epidemics and Ideas: Essays on the Historical Perception of Pestilence*, ed. Terence Ranger and Paul Slack, 203–240. Cambridge: Cambridge University Press, 1992.

Chandran, Nisha, and Samir K. Brahmachari. 'Policy as a Driver of Economic Growth: Historical Evidence from the Indian Pharmaceutical Industry'. *Current Science* 114, no. 6 (2018): 1181–93. http://dx.doi.org/10.18520/cs/v114/i06/1181-1193.

Chatterjee, Animesh. '"New Wine in New Bottles": Class Politics and the "Uneven Electrification" of Colonial India'. *History of Retailing and Consumption* 4, no .1 (2018): 94–108. https://doi.org/10.1080/2373518X.2018.1436226.

Chatterjee, D.N. *Drugs of India*. Calcutta: McBlain Books, 1934.

Chatterjee, Partha. 'Development Planning and the Indian State'. In *Politics and the State in India*, ed. Zoya Hasan, 120–5. New Delhi: Sage Publications, 2000.

– *The Nation and its Fragments: Colonial and Postcolonial Histories*. New Jersey: Princeton University Press, 1993.

– *Nationalist Thought and Colonial India: A Derivative Discourse?* Delhi: Zed Books, 1986.

Chatterjee, Ratnabali. 'The Indian Prostitute as a Colonial Subject: Bengal 1864–1883'. *Canadian Woman Studies* 13, no. 1 (1992): 51–5.

Chaudhuri, R.N., and H. Chakravarti. 'Typhus in Calcutta'. *Indian Medical Gazette* 84, no. 8 (1949): 43–51.

Chaudhuri, Rosinka. 'Modernity at Home: The Nationalization of the Indian Drawing Room, 1830–1930'. In *Interpreting Homes in South Asian Literature*, ed. M. Lal and S.P. Kumar, 221–40. Delhi: Pearson Longman, 2007.

Chaudhuri, Sudip. 'Multinationals and Monopolies: Pharmaceutical Industry in India after TRIPS'. *Economic and Political Weekly* 47, no. 12 (2012): 46–54. https://www.epw.in/journal/2012/12/special-articles/multinationals-and-monopolies.html.

– *The WTO and India's Pharmaceuticals Industry: Patent Protection, TRIPS, and Developing Countries*. New Delhi: Oxford University Press, 2005.

Chopra, R.N. 'Drug Adulteration and Spurious Drugs in India'. *The Indian Medical Gazette* 70, no. 12 (1935): 693. https://www.ncbi.nlm.nih.gov/pmc/issues/281464/#.

– 'The Drug Industry in India and its Difficulties'. *The Indian Medical Gazette* 74, no. 4 (1939): 230. https://pubmed.ncbi.nlm.nih.gov/29011753.

– 'Drug Manufacture in India During Peace and War'. *The Indian Medical Gazette* 75, no. 4 (1940): 233.

– *Indigenous Drugs of India: Their Medical and Economic Aspects*. Art Press, 1933.

– 'Some Aspects of Therapeutics in India'. *The Indian Medical Gazette* 62, no. 3 (1927): 151. https://www.ncbi.nlm.nih.gov/pmc/issues/282497/#.

Chowdhury, Subhadeep. 'Medicine and Colonial Patent Law in India: A Study of Patent Medicines and the Indian Patents and Designs Act, 1911 in Early-Twentieth-Century India'. *Journal of the History of Medicine and Allied Sciences* 75, no. 4 (2020): 408–28. https://doi.org/10.1093/jhmas/jraa027.

Chuckerbutty, S. Goodeve. 'The Present State of the Medical Profession in Bengal'. *British Medical Journal* (July 1864): 111.

Church, Roy. 'The British Market for Medicine in the Late Nineteenth Century: The Innovative Impact of SM Burroughs & Co'. *Medical History* 49, no. 3 (2005): 281–98. https://doi.org/10.1017%2Fs0025727300008887.

Cleetus, Burton. 'Subaltern Medicine and Social Mobility: The Experience of the Ezhava in Kerala'. *Indian Anthropologist* 37, no. 1 (2007): 147–72. http://www.jstor.org/stable/41920032.

Cohn, Bernard S. 'Law and the Colonial State in India'. In *History and Power in the Study of Law: New Directions in Legal Anthropology*, ed. June Starr and Jane F. Collier, 131–52. Cornell University Press, 1989. http://www.jstor.org/stable/10.7591/j.ctt207g6xn.10.

Compton, Herbert. *Indian Life in Town and Country*, London: G. Newnes, 1904.

Cook, Harold J., and Timothy D. Walker. 'Circulation of Medicine in the Early Modern Atlantic World'. *Social History of Medicine* 26, no. 3 (2013): 337–51. https://doi.org/10.1093/shm/hkt013.

Cramer, Tobias. 'Building the "World's Pharmacy": The Rise of the German Pharmaceutical Industry, 1871–1914'. *Business History Review* 89, no. 1 (2015): 43–73. https://doi.org/10.1017/s0007680515000057.

Crellin, J. K. 'Pharmaceutical History and its Sources in the Wellcome Collections. I. The Growth of Professionalism in Nineteenth-century British Pharmacy'. *Medical History* 11, no. 3 (1967): 215–27. https://doi.org/10.1017/s0025727300012321.

Cutler J.C., Johs Kvitingen, Evelyn Rose, James C. McCullough, R.B. Tampi, Sukumar Sen, Chandra Parmer, and Girdharil Lal. 'Mass Treatment of Syphilis in an Indian Province: Report of the World Health Organization Venereal Disease Demonstration Team in the Ghund Area of the Himachal Pradesh, India'. *Bull World Health Organ* 5, no. 4 (1952): 377–439. https://pubmed.ncbi.nlm.nih.gov/14935784.

da Costa, Palmira Fontes. 'Geographical Expansion and the Reconfiguration of Medical Authority: Garcia de Orta's Colloquies on the Simples and Drugs of India (1563)'. *Studies in History and Philosophy of Science Part A* 43, no. 1 (2012): 74–81. https://doi.org/10.1016/j.shpsa.2011.09.015.

Dahdah, Marine Al, Aalok Kumar, and Mathieu Quet. 'Empty Stocks and Loose Paper: Governing Access to Medicines through Informality in Northern India'. *International Sociology* 33, no. 6 (2018): 778–95. https://doi.org/10.1177%2F0268580918792779.

Dale, H. 'Science in War and Peace'. *Nature* 160 (1947): 280–3. https://doi.org/10.1038/160280a0.

Dalmia, Vasudha. *The Nationalization of Hindu Traditions: Bh ratendu Hari chandra and Nineteenth-century Banaras*. Delhi: Oxford University Press, 1999.

Dannhaeuser, Norbert. 'From the Metropolis into the Up-Country: The Stockist System in India's Developing Mass Consumer Market'. *The Journal of Developing Areas* 21, no. 3 (1987) 259–76. http://www.jstor.org/stable/4191561.

Das, Shinjini. *Vernacular Medicine in Colonial India: Family, Market and Homeopathy*. Cambridge: Cambridge University Press, 2019.

David, J., and C. Vareed. 'Deterioration of the Digitalis Glucosides in the Tropics'. *The Madras Medical Journal* 11, no. 4 (1929): 41–53.

Deb Roy, Rohan. *Malarial Subjects: Empire, Medicine and Nonhumans in British India, 1820–1909*. Cambridge: Cambridge University Press, 2017.

Deshpande, Anirudh. 'An Historical Overview of Opium Cultivation and Changing State Attitudes towards the Crop in India, 1878–2000 AD'. *Studies in History* 25, no. 1 (2009): 109–43. https://doi.org/10.1177%2F025764300902500105.

Digby, Anne. *Making a Medical Living: Doctors and Patients in the English Market for Medicine, 1720–1911*. Cambridge: Cambridge University Press, 1994.

Dorner, Zachary. *Merchants of Medicines*. Chicago: University of Chicago Press, 2020.

Drayton, Richard. *Nature's Government*. New Delhi: Orient BlackSwan, 2005.

Dutt, N.B. *Commercial Drugs of India*. Calcutta: Thacker, Spink, and Company, 1928.

Dymock, W., C.J.H. Warden, and D. Hooper. *Pharmacographia Indica: A History of the Principal Drugs of Vegetable Origin Met with in British India*. London: Kegan Paul, Trench Trübner, 1893.

Edwards, Penny. 'Bitter Pills: Colonialism, Medicine and Nationalism in Burma, 1870–1940'. *Journal of Burma Studies* 14, no. 1 (2010): 21–58. http://dx.doi.org/10.1353/jbs.2010.0005.

Eglash, Ron, ed. *Appropriating Technology: Vernacular Science and Social Power*. Minneapolis: University of Minnesota Press, 2004.

Ellis, Catriona. '"If You Cannot Feed the Body of a Child You Cannot Feed the Brain": Education and Nutrition in Late Colonial Madras'. *South Asia: Journal of South Asian Studies* 44, no. 1 (2021): 135–51. https://doi.org/10.1080/00856401.2021.1862497.

Evans, J.F., and Chunilal Bose. 'The Necessity for an Act Restricting the Free Sale of Poisons in Bengal'. In *The Scientific and other Papers of Rai Chunilal Bose Bahadur*. Calcutta: NA, 1924. https://doi.org/10.11588/xarep.00002782.

Fraser, D.A. Campbell. *The British Medical Officer's Indian Manual*. Calcutta: Wyman & Co., 1870.

Freitag, Sandria B. *Collective Action and Community: Public Arenas and the Emergence of Communalism in North India*. Berkeley: University of California Press, 1989.

Furedy, Chris. *British Tradesmen and Shopkeepers of Calcutta, 1830–1900*. Self-published, 1976.

Ganesan, Uma. 'Medicine and Modernity: The Ayurvedic Revival Movement in India, 1885–1947'. *Studies on Asia* 4, no. 1 (2010): 108–31.

Gerth, Karl. 'Consumption and Nationalism: China'. In *The Oxford Handbook of the History of Consumption*, ed. Frank Trentmann. Oxford: Oxford University Press, 2012.

Ghai, Damanjeet. 'Patent Protection and Indian Pharmaceutical Industry'. *International Journal of Pharmaceutical Sciences Review and Research* 3, no. 2 (2010): 43–8.

Ghosh, Durba. 'Whither India? 1919 and the Aftermath of the First World War'. *The Journal of Asian Studies* 78, no. 2 (2019): 389–97. http://dx.doi.org/10.1017/S0021911819000044.

Ghosh, S. 'The Scientific and Economic Importance of Research on Indian Medicinal Plants'. *The Indian Medical Gazette* 63, no. 11 (November 1928): 650–3. https://www.ncbi.nlm.nih.gov/pmc/issues/284256/#.

Gopinath, Arunima. 'Imagining Communities–Differently: Print, Language and the (Public Sphere) in Colonial Kerala'. *The Indian Economic & Social History Review* 43, no. 1 (2006): 63–76. https://doi.org/10.1177/001946460504300103.

Goswami, Omkar. 'Sahibs, Babus, and Banias: Changes in Industrial Control in Eastern India, 1918–50'. *The Journal of Asian Studies* 48, no. 2 (1989): 289–309. https://doi.org/10.2307/2057379.

Greene Willam, *The Emergence of India's Pharmaceutical Industry and Implications for the U.S. Generic Drug Market*, Office of Economics Working Paper, US International Trade Commission, May 2007.

Jeremy A. Greene, Flurin Condrau, and Siegel Watkins Elizabeth, eds. *Therapeutic Revolutions: Pharmaceuticals and Social Change in the Twentieth Century*. Chicago: University of Chicago Press, 2016.

Grove, Richard. 'Indigenous Knowledge and the Significance of South-West India for Portuguese and Dutch Constructions of Tropical Nature'. *Modern Asian Studies* 30, no. 1 (1996): 121–43. https://doi.org/10.1017/S0026749X00014104.

Gupta, Charu. 'Procreation and Pleasure: Writings of a Woman Ayurvedic Practitioner in Colonial North India'. *Studies in History* 21, no. 1 (2005): 17–44. http://dx.doi.org/10.1177/025764300502100102.

Hamied, K.A. *An Autobiography: A Life to Remember*. Bombay: Lalvani Publishing House, 1972.

Haq, M.E. 'British Narco-diplomacy, 1909–46'. In *Drugs in South Asia*. London: Palgrave Macmillan, 2000.

Hardiman, David. 'From Custom to Crime: The Politics of Drinking in Colonial South Gujarat'. In *Subaltern Studies* 4, ed. Ranajit Guha, 165–228. Delhi: Oxford University Press, 1985.

– 'Indian Medical Indigeneity: From Nationalist Assertion to the Global Market'. *Social History* 34, no. 3 (2009): 263–83. http://dx.doi.org/10.1080/03071020902975131.
– *Missionaries and their Medicine: A Christian Modernity for Tribal India*. Manchester: Manchester University Press, 2008.
– 'Purifying the Nation: The Arya Samaj in Gujarat 1895–1930'. *The Indian Economic & Social History Review* 44, no. 1 (2007): 41–65. https://doi.org/10.1177%2F001946460604400103.
Hardiman, David, and Projit Bihari Mukharji, eds. Introduction to *Medical Marginality in South Asia: Situating Subaltern Therapeutics*. London: Routledge, 2013.
Harrison, Mark. 'From Bazaar Medicine to Hospital Medicine: Calomel, India, and the British Empire, c. 1750–1800'. In *Medical Encounters in British India*, ed. Deepak Kumar and Raj Sekhar Basu, 61–79. Oxford: Oxford University Press, 2013.
– Introduction to *From Western Medicine to Global Medicine: The Hospital Beyond the West*. Edited by M. Harrison, M. Jones, and H. Sweet. Orient BlackSwan, 2009.
– *Medicine and Victory: British Military Medicine in the Second World War*. Oxford: Oxford University Press, 2004.
– *Medicine in an Age of Commerce and Empire: Britain and its Tropical Colonies 1660–1830*. Oxford: Oxford University Press, 2011.
– *Public Health in British India: Anglo-Indian Preventive Medicine 1859–1914*. Cambridge: Cambridge University Press, 1994.
– 'A Question of Locality: The Identity of Cholera in British India, 1860–1890'. In *Warm Climates and Western Medicine*, 133–59. Amsterdam: Brill, 1996.
– '"The Tender Frame of Man": Disease, Climate, and Racial Difference in India and the West Indies, 1760–1860'. *Bulletin of the History of Medicine* 70, no. 1 (1996): 68–93. https://doi.org/10.1353/bhm.1996.0038.
Haynes, Douglas E. 'Artisan Cloth-producers and the Emergence of Powerloom Manufacture in Western India 1920–1950'. *Past & Present* 172, no. 1 (2001): 170–98. https://doi.org/10.1093/past/172.1.170.
– 'Creating the Consumer? Advertising, Capitalism, and the Middle Class in Urban Western India, 1914–40'. In *Towards a History of Consumption in South Asia*, ed. D. E. Haynes, A. McGowan, T. Roy, and H. Yanagisawa, 185–223. Delhi: Oxford University Press, 2011.
– 'Masculinity, Advertising and the Reproduction of the Middle-Class Family in Western India'. In *Being Middle Class in India: A Way of Life*, ed. Henrike Donner, 23–46. London: Routledge, 2011.

– *Rhetoric and Ritual in Colonial India: The Shaping of a Public Culture in Surat City, 1852–1928*. Berkeley: University of California Press, 1991.

Haynes, Douglas E., and Abigail McGowan. Introduction to *Towards a History of Consumption in South Asia*. Edited by Douglas E. Haynes. India: Oxford University Press, 2010.

Hendriksen, Marieke M.A. 'Consumer Culture, Self-Prescription, and Status: Nineteenth-Century Medicine Chests in the Royal Navy'. *Journal of Victorian Culture* 20, no. 2 (2015): 147–67. https://doi.org/10.1080/13555502.2015.1022353.

Hervey, H.J.A. *The European in India*. London: S. Paul & Company, 1913.

Higby, Gregory J. 'Professionalism and the Nineteenth-century American Pharmacist'. *Pharmacy in History* 28, no. 3 (1986): 115–24. http://www.jstor.org/stable/41109797.

Hodges, Sarah. 'The Case of the 'Spurious Drugs Kingpin': Shifting Pills in Chennai, India'. *Critical Public Health* 29, no. 4 (2019): 473–83. https://doi.org/10.1080%2F09581596.2019.1593948.

Hogg, Francis. *Practical Remedies Chiefly Concerning the Health and Ailments of European Families in India, with Special Reference to Maternal Management and Domestic Economy*. Benares: Medical Hall Press, 1877.

Holloway, S.W.F. 'Producing Experts, Constructing Expertise: The School of Pharmacy of the Pharmaceutical Society of Great Britain, 1842–1896'. *Clio Med* 30 (1995): 116–40.

Inamdar, Nikhil. *Rokda: How Banias Do Business*. Random House India, 2014.

Isaacs, Jeremy D. 'DD Cunningham and the Aetiology of Cholera in British India, 1869–1897'. *Medical History* 42, no. 3 (1998): 279–305. doi:10.1017/S0025727300063997.

Islam, Nazrul. 'Indigenous Medicine as Commodity: Local Reach of Ayurveda in Modern India'. *Current Sociology* 58, no. 5 (2010): 777–98. https://doi.org/10.1177%2F0011392110372739.

Iswariah, V. 'The Pharmacy Bill'. *Indian Medical Gazette* (August 1946): 334. https://www.ncbi.nlm.nih.gov/pmc/issues/284284/#.

Jeffery, Roger. 'Recognizing India's Doctors: The Institutionalization of Medical Dependency, 1918–39'. *Modern Asian Studies* 13, no. 2 (1979): 301–26. http://www.jstor.org/stable/312127.

Jenkinson, Jacqueline. 'A "Crutch to Assist in Gaining an Honest Living": Dispensary Shopkeeping by Scottish General Practitioners and the Responses of the British Medical Elite, ca. 1852–1911'. *Bulletin of the History of Medicine* 86, no. 1 (2012): 1–36. https://doi.org/10.1353/bhm.2012.0008.

Johnson, Ryan. 'Commodity Culture: Tropical Health and Hygiene in the British Empire'. *Endeavour* 32, no. 2 (2008): 70–4. https://doi.org/10.1353/bhm.0.0252.

Johnson, Ryan, and Amna Khalid. *Public Health in the British Empire: Intermediaries, Subordinates, and the Practice of Public Health, 1850–1960*. London: Routledge, 2012.

Joshi, Sanjay, ed. *The Middle Class in Colonial India*. Oxford: Oxford University Press, 2010.

Kaminsky, Arnold P. 'Morality Legislation and British Troops in Late Nineteenth-century India'. *The Journal of Military History* 43, no. 2 (1979): 78. https://doi.org/10.2307/1986662.

Kamra, Sukeshi. 'Law and Radical Rhetoric in British India: The 1897 Trial of Bal Gangadhar Tilak'. *South Asia: Journal of South Asian Studies* 39, no. 3 (2016): 546–59. https://doi.org/10.1080/00856401.2016.1196529.

Kanny Lall Dey, Rai Bahadur. 'Presidential Address, Section of Pharmacology'. *Indian Medical Gazette* 30, no. 1 (January 1895): 25–8. https://www.ncbi.nlm.nih.gov/pmc/issues/280450/#.

Kaviraj, Sudipta. 'Development Planning in the Indian State'. In *Politics and the State in India*, ed. Zoya Hassan. Delhi: Sage Publications, 2000.

Keene, R.G. *Handbook for Visitors: Allahabad, Cawnpore and Lucknow*. Calcutta: Thacker, Spink and Company, 1896.

Kennedy, Dane. 'The Perils of the Midday Sun: Climatic Anxieties in the Colonial Tropics'. In *Imperialism and the Natural World*. Manchester: Manchester University Press, 2017.

Khanna, Aman Raj, and Hemant Krishan Singh. *India's IPR Regime: Reconciling Affordable Access with Patent Protection*. Indian Council for Research on International Economic Relations 2015.

Kidambi, Prashant. '"An infection of locality": Plague, Pythogenesis and the Poor in Bombay, c. 1896–1905'. *Urban History* 31 no. 2 (2004): 249–67. http://dx.doi.org/10.1017/S0963926804002135.

Kim, Hoi-Eun. 'Adulterated Intermediaries: Peddlers, Pharmacists, and the Patent Medicine Industry in Colonial Korea (1910–1945)'. *Enterprise & Society* 20, no. 4 (2019): 939–77. doi:10.1017/eso.2019.14.

Krishna, V.V. 'Organisation of Scientific Research: The Early History of the CSIR, 1934-47'. In *Science and Modern India: An Institutional History, 1784–1947*, ed. Uma Dasgupta. Delhi: Pearson Longman, 2011.

Kumar, A.N. Arun, Geeta Joshi, and H.Y. Mohan Ram. 'Sandalwood: History, Uses, Present Status and the Future'. *Current Science* 103, no. 12 (2012): 1408–16.

Kumar, Anil. 'The Indian Drug Industry under the Raj, 1860–1920'. In *Health, Medicine and Empire: Perspectives on Colonial India*, ed. Biswamoy Pati and Mark Harrison, 356–85. Hyderabad: Orient Longman, 2001.

Kumar, Arun. 'Skilling and Its Histories: Labour Market, Technical Knowledge and the Making of Skilled Workers in Colonial India (1880–1910)'. *Journal of South Asian Development* 13, no. 3 (2019): 249–71. https://doi.org/10.1177%2F0973174118810050.

Kumar, Deepak. 'Reconstructing India: Disunity in the Science and Technology for Development Discourse, 1900–1947'. *Osiris* 15, no. 1 (2000): 241–57. http://dx.doi.org/10.1086/649329.

– 'Unequal Contenders, Uneven Ground: Medical Encounters in British India, 1820–1920'. In *Western Medicine as Contested Knowledge*, ed. Bridie Andrews and Andrew Cunningham. Manchester: Manchester University Press, 2017.

Lal, Maneesha. 'The Politics of Gender and Medicine in Colonial India: The Countess of Dufferin's Fund, 1885–1888'. *Bulletin of the History of Medicine* 68, no. 1 (1994): 29–66. http://www.jstor.org/stable/44451545.

Lambert, Helen. 'Medical Pluralism and Medical Marginality: Bone Doctors and the Selective Legitimation of Therapeutic Expertise in India'. *Social Science & Medicine* 74, no. 7 (2012): 1029–36. https://doi.org/10.1016/j.socscimed.2011.12.024.

Lang, Sean. 'Drop the Demon Dai: Maternal Mortality and the State in Colonial Madras, 1840–1875'. *Social History of Medicine* 18, no. 3 (2005): 357–78. http://dx.doi.org/10.1093/shm/hki052.

Legg, Stephen. '"The Life of Individuals as Well as of Nations": International Law and the League of Nations' Anti-trafficking Governmentalities'. *Leiden Journal of International Law* 25, no. 3 (2012): 647–64. DOI:10.1017/S0922156512000325.

– 'Stimulation, Segregation and Scandal: Geographies of Prostitution Regulation in British India, Between Registration (1888) and Suppression (1923)'. *Modern Asian Studies* 46, no. 6 (2012): 1459–505. https://doi.org/10.1017/s0026749x11000503.

Lei, Sean Hsiang-lin. *Neither Donkey nor Horse: Medicine in the Struggle over China's Modernity*. Chicago: University of Chicago Press, 2014.

Lesch, John E. *The First Miracle Drugs: How the Sulfa Drugs Transformed Medicine*. New York: Oxford University Press, 2007.

Leslie, Charles, ed. 'The Ambiguities of Medical Revivalism in Modern India'. In *Asian Medical Systems: A Comparative Study*, 356–67. Berkeley: University of California Press, 1976.

– 'Pluralism and Integration in the Indian and Chinese Medical Systems'. In *Medicine in Chinese Cultures: Comparative Cross-Cultural Studies of Health Care in Chinese and Other Societies*, ed. Arthur Kleinman et al., 401–17. USA: University Press of the Pacific, 2005.

Levine, Philippa. 'Rereading the 1890s: Venereal Disease as "Constitutional Crisis" in Britain and British India'. *The Journal of Asian Studies* 55, no. 3 (1996): 585–612. https://doi.org/10.2307/2646447.

– 'Venereal Disease, Prostitution, and the Politics of Empire: The Case of British India'. *Journal of the History of Sexuality* 4, no. 4 (1994): 579–602.

Liebenau, Jonathan. 'Ethical Business: The Formation of the Pharmaceutical Industry in Britain, Germany, and the United States Before 1914'. *Business History* 30, no. 1 (1988): 116–29. https://doi.org/10.1080/00076798800000007.

Livingstone, David N. 'Tropical Climate and Moral Hygiene: The Anatomy of a Victorian Debate'. *The British Journal for the History of Science* 32, no. 1 (1999): 93–110. http://www.jstor.org/stable/4027971.

Loeb, Lori. 'Doctors and Patent Medicines in Modern Britain: Professionalism and Consumerism'. *Albion: A Quarterly Journal Concerned with British Studies* 33, no. 3 (2001): 404–25. https://doi.org/10.2307/4053198.

Löfgren, H., ed. *The Politics of the Pharmaceutical Industry and Access to Medicines: World Pharmacy and India*. London and New York: Routledge, 2018.

Mackintosh, Alan. 'The Legacy of the Patent Medicines Industry'. In *The Patent Medicines Industry in Georgian England*, 261–74. Palgrave Macmillan, 2018.

Mair, R.S., and Edmund C.P. Hull. *The European in India; Or, Anglo-Indian's Vade-Mecum*. London: Henry S. King, 1871.

Malleck, D. Professionalism and the Boundaries of Control: Pharmacists, Physicians and Dangerous Substances in Canada, 1840–1908. *Medical History* 48, no. 2 (2004): 175–98. https://doi.org/10.1017%2Fs0025727300007389.

Mani, Lata. 'Contentious Traditions: The Debate on Sati in Colonial India'. *Cultural Critique*, no. 7 (1987): 119–56. https://doi.org/10.2307/1354153.

Mantena, Rama Sundari. 'Vernacular Publics and Political Modernity: Language and Progress in Colonial South India'. *Modern Asian Studies* 47, no. 5 (2013): 1678–1705. http://www.jstor.org/stable/24494224.

Marland, Hilary, and Adams Jane. 'Hydropathy at Home: The Water Cure and Domestic Healing in Mid-Nineteenth-Century Britain'. *Bulletin of the History of Medicine* 83, no. 3 (2009): 499. https://doi.org/10.1353/bhm.0.0251.

Mazumdar, Madhumita. 'Reflecting on Chemical Education: Nilratan Dhar and the Legacy of PC Ray'. *Indian Journal of History of Science* 53, no. 4 (2018): T94–T99. DOI: 10.16943/ijhs/2018/v53i4/49531.

McRobert, George R. 'The Position of Medical Science in India'. *The Indian Medical Gazette* 79, no. 12 (December 1944): 607–11. https://www.ncbi.nlm.nih.gov/pmc/issues/283478/#.

Mehta, Makrand. 1984. 'Institution Building in Princely India: A Case Study of the Polytechnic Institute, Baroda, 1890–18962'. Paper presented at *Proceedings of the Indian History Congress* 45, 1984.

Metcalf, Barbara D. 'Nationalist Muslims in British India: The Case of Hakim Ajmal Khan'. *Modern Asian Studies* 19, no.1 (1985): 1–28. http://www.jstor.org/stable/312319.

Michelutti, Lucia. '"We are Kshatriyas but we Behave like Vaishyas": Diet and Muscular Politics Among a Community of Yadavs in North India'. *South Asia: Journal of South Asian Studies* 31, no.1 (2008): 76–95. https://doi.org/10.1080/00856400701874726.

Mills, James H. 'Cocaine and the British Empire: The Drug and the Diplomats at the Hague Opium Conference, 1911–12'. *The Journal of Imperial and Commonwealth History* 42, no. 3 (2014): 400–19. https://doi.org/10.1080/03086534.2014.894701.

– 'Drugs, Consumption, and Supply in Asia: The Case of Cocaine in Colonial India, c. 1900–c. 1930'. *The Journal of Asian Studies* 66, no. 2 (2007): 345–62. http://www.jstor.org/stable/20203161.

Mishra, Saurabh. *Beastly Encounters of the Raj: Livelihoods, Livestock and Veterinary Health in North India, 1790–1920*. Manchester: Manchester University Press, 2015.

– *Pilgrimage, Politics, and Pestilence: The Haj from the Indian Subcontinent, 1860–1920*. Delhi: Oxford University Press, 2010.

Monnais, Laurence. *The Colonial Life of Pharmaceuticals*. Cambridge: Cambridge University Press, 2019.

Mukharji, Projit Bihari. 'Baidya-as-Technology: From Diagnosis to Pharmacy in a Bottle'. In *Doctoring Traditions: Ayurveda, Small Technologies and Braided Sciences*, 227–56. Chicago: University of Chicago Press, 2016.

– *Doctoring Traditions: Ayurveda, Small Technologies, and Braided Sciences*. Chicago: Chicago University Press, 2016.

– *Nationalizing the Body: The Medical Market, Print, and Daktari Medicine*. London and New York: Anthem Press, 2009.

– 'Pharmacology, "Indigenous Knowledge", Nationalism: A Few Words from the Epitaph of Subaltern Science'. In *The Social History of Health and Medicine in Colonial India*, ed. B. Pati and M. Harrison, 195–212. London: Routledge, 2009.

– 'Vishalyakarani as Eupatorium Ayapana: Retro-Botanizing, Embedded Traditions, and Multiple Historicities of Plants in Colonial Bengal, 1890–1940'. *The Journal of Asian Studies* 73, no. 1 (2014): 65–87. http://dx.doi.org/10.1017/S0021911813001733.

– 'What's in a Name?: The Crisis of Botanical Identification and the Production of "Economic Man"'. *Social Scientist* 33, no. 5/6 (2005): 3–25.

Mukherjee, Janam. *Hungry Bengal: War, Famine, and the End of Empire*. Oxford: Oxford University Press, 2015.

Mukhopadhyay, Bhaskar. 'Between Elite Hysteria and Subaltern Carnivalesque: The Politics of Street-Food in the City of Calcutta'. *South Asia Research* 24, no. 1 (2004): 37–50. https://doi.org/10.1177%2F0262728004042762.

Muraleedharan, V.R. 'Professionalising Medical Practice in Colonial South-India'. *Economic and Political Weekly* 27, no. 4 (1992): PE27–PE37. http://www.jstor.org/stable/4397525.

– 'Quinine (Cinchona) and the Incurable Malaria: India c. 1900–1930s'. *Parassitologia* 42, no. 1–2 (2000): 91–100.

Nair, Janaki. 'Modernity and "Publicness": The Career of the Mysore Matha, 1880–1940'. *The Indian Economic & Social History Review* 57, no. 1 (2020): 5–29. https://doi.org/10.1177%2F0019464619892891.

Nanavati, Manilal B. *Notes on Industrial Development in the Baroda State*. Baroda: Baroda Printing Works, 1916.

Naraindas, Harish. 'Care, Welfare, and Treason: The Advent of Vaccination in the 19th Century,' *Contributions to Indian Sociology* 32, no. 1 (1998): 67–96. https://doi.org/10.1177%2F006996679803200104.

Naregal, Veena. *Language Politics, Elites, and the Public Sphere: Western India under Colonialism*. New Delhi: Permanent Black, 2001.

Nayar, Baldev Raj. 'Nationalist Planning for Autarky and State Hegemony: Development Strategy Uder Nehru'. *Indian Economic Review* 32, no. 1 (1997): 13–38. http://www.jstor.org/stable/24010467.

Nijhawan, Shobna. 'Cumin, Capsules, and Colonialism: "Real" and "Imagined" Medical Encounters in the Hindi Literary Sphere'. *Asian Medicine* 13, no. 1–2 (2018): 170–97. https://doi.org/10.1163/15734218-12341412.

Oberoi, Harjot Singh. 'The Worship of Pir Sakhi Sarvar: Illness, Healing and Popular Culture in the Punjab'. *Studies in History* 3, no. 1 (1987): 29–55. https://doi.org/10.1177%2F025764308700300104.

Ombongi, Kenneth. 'The Historical Interface between the State and Medical Science in Africa: Kenya's Case'. In *Evidence, Ethos and Experiment: The Anthropology of Medical Research in Africa*, 353–72. New York and Oxford: Bergham Books, 2011.

O'Meara, E.J. *Medical Guide for India and Book of Prescriptions*. London: Butterworth and Co., 1920.

Orsini, Francesca. *The Hindi Public Sphere 1920–1940: Language and Literature in the Age of Nationalism*. New Delhi: Oxford University Press, 2009.

O'Shaughnessy, William Brooke. *The Bengal Dispensatory & Companion to the Pharmacopoeia: Chiefly Compiled from the Works of Roxburgh, Wallich, Ainslie [etc.]*. London: W.H. Allen & Co, 1842.

Osseo-Asare, Abena Dove. *Bitter Roots: The Search for Healing Plants in Africa*. Chicago: University of Chicago Press, 2014.

Panikkar, K.N. 'Indigenous Medicine and Cultural Hegemony: A Study of the Revitalization Movement in Keralam'. *Studies in History* 8, no. 2 (1992): 283–308. https://doi.org/10.1177%2F025764309200800206.

Pearn, John. '"Where There is No Doctor": Self-Help and Pre-Hospital Care in Colonial Australia'. *Health and History* 14, no. 2 (2012): 162–180. http://dx.doi.org/10.5401/healthhist.14.2.0162.

Peers, Douglas M. 'Soldiers, Surgeons and the Campaigns to Combat Sexually Transmitted Diseases in Colonial India, 1805–1860'. *Medical History* 42, no. 2 (1998): 137–160. DOI:10.1017/S0025727300063651.

Perkins, C. Ryan. 'From the Me fil to the Printed Word: Public Debate and Discourse in Late Colonial India'. *The Indian Economic & Social History Review* 50, no. 1 (2013): 47–76. https://doi.org/10.1177/0019464612474169.

Pharmacopoeia of India, Delhi: Manager of Publications, 1955.

Phipson, E.S. '"Patent" Medicines, the Public, and the Doctor'. *The Indian Medical Gazette* 74, no. 2 (1939): 98.

Podolsky, Scott H. *The Antibiotic Era: Reform, Resistance, and the Pursuit of a Rational Therapeutics*. Baltimore: Johns Hopkins Press, 2015.

Pols, Hans. 'Notes from Batavia, the Europeans' Graveyard: The Nineteenth-century Debate on Acclimatization in the Dutch East Indies'. *Journal of the History of Medicine and Allied Sciences* 67, no. 1 (2012): 120–148. https://doi.org/10.1093/jhmas/jrr004.

Pordié Laurent, and Gaudillière Jean-Paul. 'The Reformulation Regime in Drug Discovery: Revisiting Polyherbals and Property Rights in the Ayurvedic Industry'. *East Asian Science, Technology and Society: An International Journal* 8, no. 1 (2014): 57–79. http://dx.doi.org/10.1215/18752160-2406053.

Roy, Porter. *Health for Sale: Quackery in England 1660–1850*. Manchester and New York: Manchester University Press, 1989.

Prasad, Srirupa. 'Crisis, Identity, and Social Distinction: Cultural Politics of Food, Taste, and Consumption in Late Colonial Bengal'. *Journal of Historical Sociology* 19, no. 3 (2006): 245–65. https://doi.org/10.1111/j.1467-6443.2006.00281.x.

– *Cultural Politics of Hygiene in India, 1890–1940: Contagions of Feeling*. Springer, 2015.

Prashad, Vijay. 'Marks of Capital: Colonialism and the Sweepers of Delhi'. *International Review of Social History* 40, no. 1 (1995): 1–30. doi:10.1017/S0020859000113008.

Qadeer, Imrana. 'Health Planning in India: Some Lessons from the Past'. *Social Scientist* 36, no. 5/6 (2008): 51–75. http://www.jstor.org/stable/27644278.

Quaiser, Neshat. 'Colonial Politics of Medicine and Popular Unani Resistance'. *Indian Horizons* 47, no. 2 (2000): 29–42.

– 'Politics, Culture and Colonialism: Unani's Debate with Doctory'. In *Health, Medicine and Empire: Perspectives on Colonial India*, ed. Biswamoy Pati and Mark Harrison, 317–55. Hyderabad: Orient Longman, 2001.

– 'Science, Institution and Colonialism: Tibbiya College of Delhi, 1889–1947'. In *Science and Modern India: An Institutional History, c 1947*, ed. Uma das Gupta, 523–61. Delhi: Pearson, 2010.

Quirke, Viviane, and Jean-Paul Gaudillière. 'The Era of Biomedicine: Science, Medicine, and Public Health in Britain and France after the Second World War'. *Medical History* 52, no. 4 (2008): 441–52. https://doi.org/10.1017%2Fs002572730000017x.

Rai, Saurav Kumar. 'Invoking "Hindu" Ayurveda: Communalisation of the Late Colonial Ayurvedic Discourse'. *The Indian Economic & Social History Review* 56, no. 4 (2019): 411–26. https://doi.org/10.1177%2F0019464619873820.

Raina, Dhruv, and S. Irfan Habib. 'Technical Institutes in Colonial India Kala Bhavan, Baroda (1890–1990)'. *Economic and Political Weekly* 26 (1991): 2619–24.

Rajadhyaksha, Niranjan. 'The Long Road to Indian Economic Planning (until 1950)'. In *Planning in the 20th Century and Beyond: India's Planning Commission and the NITI Aayog*, ed. Santosh Mehrotra and Sylvie Guichard, 43–60. Cambridge University Press, 2020.

Ramanna, Mridula 'Systems of Medicine: Issues and Responses in Bombay Presidency'. *Economic and Political Weekly* 41, 29 (2006): 3221–6. http://dx.doi.org/10.2307/4418477.

– *Western Medicine and Public Health in Colonial Bombay, 1845–1895*. New Delhi: Orient Blackswan, 2002.

Ramasubban, Radhika. 'Public Health in British India, 1857–1900'. In *Disease, Medicine, and Empire: Perspectives on Western Medicine and the Experience of European Expansion*, ed. R. McLeod and M. Lewis, 38–60. London: Routledge, 2022.

Rao, Mohan et al. 'India: Towards Universal Health Coverage 5 Human Resources for Health in India'. *Lancet* 377 (2011): 587–98. DOI:10.1016/S0140- 6736(10)61888-0.

Rao, Mohan, Krishna D. Rao, AK Shiva Kumar, Mirai Chatterjee, and Thiagarajan

Sundararaman. 'Human Resources for Health in India'. *The Lancet* 377, no. 9765 (2011): 587–98. https://doi.org/10.1016/s0140-6736(10)61888-0.

Rao, Tirumal B. 'A Plea for the Study of Indigenous Medicine by the Indian Allopathist'. *The Madras Medical Journal* 1, no. 4 (1918): 187–94.

Ray, Utsa. 'The Body and its Purity: Detary Politics in Colonial Bengal'. *The Indian Economic & Social History Review* 50, no. 4 (2013): 395–421. https://doi.org/10.1177%2F0019464613502413.

Renford, R. *The Non-official British in India to 1920*. Delhi: OUP India Press, 1987.

Richards, John F. 'The Opium Industry in British India'. *The Indian Economic & Social History Review* 39, nos 2–3 (2002): 149–80. https://doi.org/10.1177%2F001946460203900203.

Roberts, Michael J.D. 'The Politics of Professionalization: MPs, Medical Men, and the 1858 Medical Act'. *Medical History* 53, no. 1 (2009): 37–56. https://doi.org/10.1017/s0025727300003306.

Roger, Jeffrey. *The Politics of Health in India*. Berkeley: University of California Press, 1988.

Rosenberg, Charles E. 'The Therapeutic Revolution: Medicine, Meaning, and Social Change in Nineteenth-century America'. *Perspectives in Biology and Medicine* 20, no. 4 (1977): 485–506. https://doi.org/10.1353/pbm.1977.0040.

Roy, Church, and E.M. Tansey. *Burroughs, Wellcome & Co.: Knowledge, Trust, Profit and the Transformation of the British Pharmaceutical Industry, 1880–1940*. Lancaster: Crucible Books, 2007.

Roy, Kaushik. 'Equipping Leviathan: Ordnance Factories of British India, 1859–1913'. *War in History* 10, no. 4 (2003): 398–423. https://doi.org/10.1191/0968344503wh278oa.

Roy, P. 'Meat–Eating, Masculinity, and Renunciation in India: A Gandhian Grammar of Diet'. *Gender & History* 14, no. 1 (2002): 62–91. http://dx.doi.org/10.1111/1468-0424.00252.

Roy, Tirthankar. 'The Origins of Import Substituting Industrialization in India'. *Economic History of Developing Regions* 32, no. 1 (2017): 71–95. https://doi.org/10.1080/20780389.2017.1292460.

– *Traditional Industry in the Economy of Colonial India*. Vol. 5. Cambridge: Cambridge University Press, 1999.

Royle, J.F. *An Essay on the Antiquity of Hindoo Medicine: Including an Introductory Lecture to the Course of Materia Medica and Therapeutics, Delivered at King's College*. London: W.H. Allen, J. Churchill, 1837.

– *A Manual of Materia Medica and Therapeutics: Including the Preparations of the Pharmacopœias of London, Edinburgh and Dublin*. London: John Churchill, 1847.

Saha, Ranjana. 'Milk, Mothering & Meanings: Infant Feeding in Colonial Bengal'. In *Women's Studies International Forum* 60 (2017): 97–110. https://doi.org/10.1016/j.wsif.2016.11.002.

Saha, Shuvashis, and Md Hossain. 'Evaluation of Medicines Dispensing Pattern of Private Pharmacies in Rajshahi, Bangladesh'. BMC *Health Services Research* 17, no. 1 (2017): 1–8. https://doi.org/10.1186/s12913-017-2072-z.

Sarkar, Sumit. *Swadeshi Movement in Bengal,1903–1908*. Ranikhet: Permanent Black, 2011.

Sarkar, Suvobrata. 'In Pursuit of Laxmi: Entrepreneurship, Industry and Technology in Colonial Bengal'. *Archív Orientalní* 82, no. 2 (2014).

Scroop, Daniel. 'A Faded Passion? Estes Kefauver and the Senate Subcommittee on Antitrust and Monopoly'. *Business and Economic History On-Line* 5 (2007).

Sehrawat, Samiksha. *Colonial Medical Care in North India: Gender, State and Society c. 1840–1920*. Delhi: Oxford University Press, 2013.

– 'Feminising Empire: The Association of Medical Women in India and the Campaign to Found a Women's Medical Service'. *Social Scientist* 41, no. 5/6 (2013): 65–81.

Selvanayagam, A. 'Pharmacy in Madras-Then and Now'. *The Pharmacist*, no. 1 (1 July 1939): 15–19.

Sen, Anuradha Roy. 'Imperial Policy and Travails of Indigenous Enterprise: A Study in Bengal Chemical Pharmaceutical Works'. JSIR 58, no. 2 (1999).

Sen, Srabani. 'The Beginning of Biochemical Researches in India-A Historical Perspective'. IJHS 37, no. 3 (2002): 347–65.

Shah, M.H. *Baroda by Decades*. Baroda: Self Published, 1942.

Sharma, Madhuri. 'Creating a Consumer: Exploring Medical Advertisements in Colonial India'. In *The Social History of Health and Medicine in Colonial India*, ed. B. Pati and M. Harrison, 213–28. London and New York: Routledge, 2011.

– *Indigenous and Western Medicine in Colonial India*. Delhi: Foundation Books, 2012.

Shiva, Vandana. 'North South Conflicts in Intellectual Property Rights'. *A Journal of Social Justice* 12, no. 4 (2000): 501–8. https://doi.org/10.1080/10402650020014573.

Shukla, Nitin, and Tanushree Sangal. 'Generic Drug Industry in India: The Counterfeit Spin'. *Journal of Intellectual Property Rights* 14, no. 3 (2009): 236–40.

Simmons, Anna. 'From Purgatives and Powders to Fulminate and Factories: Archives and Sources Regarding the Society of Apothecaries' Drug Supply to India, c. 1703–1882'. *Pharmaceutical Historian* 51, no. 2 (2021): 41–50.

– 'Stills, Status, Stocks and Science: The Laboratories at Apothecaries' Hall in the

Nineteenth Century'. *Ambix* 61, no. 2 (2014): 141–61. https://doi.org/10.1179/0002698014z.00000000050.

Singh, Harkishan. 'India's Medico-Pharmaceutical Inheritance from the Colonial Period'. *Pharmacy in History* 56, no. 3–4 (2014): 90–5. https://doi.org/10.26506/pharmhist.56.3-4.0090.

– 'Tribhovandas Kalyandas Gajjar (1863–1920) – Pioneer Industrial Chemist of India'. *Indian Journal of History of Science* 45, no. 3 (2010): 419–29.

Sinha, Mrinalini. *Colonial Masculinity: The 'Manly Englishman' and the 'Effeminate Bengali' in the Late Nineteenth Century*. Manchester: Manchester University Press, 2017.

Sivaramakrishnan, Kavita. *Old Potions, New Bottles*. Hyderabad: Orient Longman, 2006.

Sprawson, C.A. *Moore's Manual of Family Medicine and Hygiene for India*. 8th ed. London: J.A. Churchill, 1916.

Sreenivasan, A. 'Pharmacy and Drug Legislation in India'. *Current Science* 14, no. 3 (1945): 63–4. www.jstor.org/stable/24209041.

Stepan, Nancy. *Picturing Tropical Nature*. Cornell University Press, 2001.

Taggart, Harold F. 'Sealing on St George Island and Its Ecological Implications'. *Pacific Historical Review* 28, no. 3 (1959): 351–60. https://doi.org/10.2307/3636134.

Tandon, Nidhi. 'Growth of Advertising Industry in India'. *International Journal of Recent Scientific Research* 9, no. 1 (2018): 23622–5. http://dx.doi.org/10.24327/ijrsr.2018.0901.1502.

Tansey, Elizabeth M. 'Medicines and Men: Burroughs, Wellcome & Co, and the British Drug Industry Before the Second World War'. *Journal of the Royal Society of Medicine* 95, no. 8 (2002): 411–16. https://doi.org/10.1258%2Fjrsm.95.8.411.

Thakur, Dinesh. 'Ranbaxy Was Never the Exception'. *Economic & Political Weekly* 55, no. 7 (2020): 59.

Tilley, Helen. 'Global Histories, Vernacular Science, and African Genealogies; or, is the History of Science Ready for the World?' *Isis* 101, no. 1 (2010): 110–19. https://doi.org/10.1086/652692.

Tripathi, Dwijendra. '"Colonial Syndrome' and Technology Choices in Indian Industry'. In *Chinese and Indian Business*, 121–41. Brill, 2010.

Tulasi, G. Krishna, and B. Subba Rao. 'A Detailed Study of Patent System for Protection of Inventions'. *Indian Journal of Pharmaceutical Sciences* 70, no. 5 (2008): 547–54. https://doi.org/10.4103%2F0250-474X.45390.

Tuteja, K.L. 'Jallianwala Bagh: A Critical Juncture in the Indian National Movement'. *Social Scientist* 25, no. 1/2 (1997): 25–61. https://doi.org/10.2307/3517759.

Tyabji, Nasir. *Colonialism, Chemical Technology and Industry in Southern India, 1880–1937*. Delhi: Oxford University Press, 1995.

– 'Gaining Technical Know-How in an Unequal World: Penicillin Manufacture in Nehru's India'. *Technology and Culture* 45, no. 2 (2004): 331–49. www.jstor.org/stable/40060744.

– 'Negotiating Nonalignment: Dilemmas Attendant on Initiating Pharmaceutical Production in India'. *Technology and Culture* 53, no. 1 (2012): 37–60. www.jstor.org/stable/41475456.

van der Geest, Sjaak, and Susan Reynolds Whyte, eds. *The Context of Medicines in Developing Countries: Studies in Pharmaceutical Anthropology*. Amsterdam: Het Spinhuis Publishers, 1998.

Wadman, Meredith. 'Falsified Data Gets India's Largest Generic Drug-maker into Trouble'. *Nature* (2009). https://doi.org/10.1038/news.2009.130.

Wallis, Patrick. 'Consumption, Retailing, and Medicine in Early modern London'. *The Economic History Review* 61, no. 1 (2008): 26–53. http://www.jstor.org/stable/40057555.

– 'Exotic Drugs and English Medicine: England's Drug Trade, c. 1550–c. 1800'. *Social History of Medicine* 25, no. 1 (2011): 20–46.

Waring, Edward John. *Pharmacopœia of India: Prepared Under the Authority of Her Majesty's Secretary of State for India in Council*. WH Allen [for the India Office], 1868.

– *Remarks on the Uses of some Bazaar Medicines, and on a Few of the Common Indigenous Plants of India, According to European Practice*. Trabancore: Sircar Press, 1860.

Warner, J.H. *The Therapeutic Perspective: Medical Practice, Knowledge, and Identity in America, 1820–1885*. Princeton University Press, 1997.

Warner, John Harley. 'Physiological Theory and Therapeutic Explanation in the 1860s: The British Debate on the Medical Use of Alcohol'. *Bulletin of the History of Medicine* 54, no. 2 (1980): 235–57. http://www.jstor.org/stable/44442950.

Watts, Sheldon. 'Cholera and the Maritime Environment of Great Britain, India and the Suez Canal: 1866–1883'. *International Journal of Environmental Studies* 63, no. 1 (2006): 19–38. https://doi.org/10.1080/00207230500505122.

– 'From Rapid Change to Stasis: Official Responses to Cholera in British-ruled India and Egypt: 1860 to c. 1921'. *Journal of World History* (2001): 321–74. http://www.jstor.org/stable/20078912.

Whyte, Susan Reynolds, Sjaak van der Geest, and Anita Hardon, 'Social Lives of Medicine'. *Social Anthropology* 12, no. 2 (2002): 247–8. http://dx.doi.org/10.1017/S0964028204320586.

Winstanley, Peter. 'This World: Bad Medicine'. *British Medical Journal* 331, no. 7509 (2005): 165. https://doi.org/10.1136/bmj.331.7509.165.

Winter, Alison. 'Ethereal Epidemic: Mesmerism and the Introduction of Inhalation Anaesthesia to early Victorian London'. *Social History of Medicine* 4, no. 1 (1991): 1–27. https://doi.org/10.1093/shm/4.1.1.

Winterbottom, Anna. 'Becoming "Traditional": A Transnational History of Neem and Biopiracy Discourse'. *Osiris* 36 (2021): 262–83. https://doi.org/10.1086/713897.

Winterbottom, Anna E. 'Of the China Root: a Case Study of the Early Modern Circulation of Materia Medica'. *Social History of Medicine* 28, no. 1 (2014): 22–44. http://dx.doi.org/10.1093/shm/hku068.

Worboys, Michael. 'The Discovery of Colonial Malnutrition between the Wars'. In *Imperial Medicine and Indigenous Societies*, 208–25. Manchester: Manchester University Press, 1988.

Wujastyk, Dominik. 'Government Policy on Ayurveda in the Twentieth Century'. In *Modern and Global Ayurveda: Pluralism and Paradigms*, ed. Dagmar Wujastyk and Frederick M. Smith, 43–71. Albany: State University of New York Press, 2008.

Yalland, Zoe. *Boxwallahs: The British in Cawnpore 1857–1901*. Norwich: Michael Russell Publishing, 1994.

Yang, Timothy. 'Selling an Imperial Dream: Japanese Pharmaceuticals, National Power, and the Science of Quinine Self-Sufficiency'. *East Asian Science, Technology and Society: An International Journal* 6, no. 1 (2012): 101–25. https://doi.org/10.1215/18752160-1506520.

Young, James Harvey. 'Patent Medicines: An Early Example of Competitive Marketing'. *The Journal of Economic History* 20, no. 4 (1960): 648–56. doi:10.1017/S002205070 0109933.

– *The Toadstool Millionaires: A Social History of Patent Medicines in America before Federal Regulation*. Princeton: Princeton University Press, 2015.

Zandu Pharmaceutical Works Limited Bombay Suchipatra: Dar ni Avritti [Index and List of Prices], Bombay 1937.

Unpublished Thesis

Khan, Azhar Ali. 'Food Adulteration in India: An Appraisal under the Indian Legal System'. Diss., Aligarh Muslim University, 1992.

Mukherjee, Abhijit. 'Natural Science in Colonial Context: The Calcutta Botanic

Garden and the Agri-Horticultural Society of India, 1787–1870'. PhD diss., Jadavpur University, 1996.

Index